Praise for *DIY Sourdough*

If you have been intimidated by the idea of fermenting your own sourdough culture, John and Jessica take all the guesswork out of the process! Step by step, they guide you through selecting the right equipment and choosing the highest quality ingredients so that you may enjoy delicious, nutritious sourdough family favorites such as English muffins and cinnamon raisin bread right in the comfort of your own home. Grab this book for your favorite fresh bread enthusiast and you may be rewarded with a homemade loaf!

HANNAH CRUM co-author, *The Big Book of Kombucha*

Time to shut down your Pinterest account and get back to the basics! With the plethora of sourdough information out there, both on the internet and in books, it can be easy to get overwhelmed by this seemingly mystical process. People have been fermenting grains, baking bread, and keeping sourdough starters alive for millennia using very simple, basic techniques. John and Jessica Moody bring back the simplicity by demonstrating in clear terms how a busy homesteading family, be they rural or urban, can bake a wide range of sourdough-based baked products with ease. To boot, *DIY Sourdough* will provide you with myriad recipes for feeding your family healthy, digestible baked products for breakfast, lunch, dinner, and in-between. Sourdough needn't be time-consuming or complicated, but once you start trying these recipes out, you may very well want to re-open that Pinterest account to show your followers the nourishing baked goods you've been creating with ease!

JEREME ZIMMERMAN author, *Make Mead Like a Viking* and *Brew Beer Like a Yeti*

This clear, simple guide is written with humility and successfully explains why and how whole grains, and the fermented starters made from them, can become a healthy staple for breads, crackers, and more. Whole grain sourdough starters are different; they take time and care. Even those successful bakers who ferment starters using conventional flours can now convert to home-milled, whole grain starters with ease. Family bakers will benefit from the experience-driven timetables and recipes that keep the carbs coming without much of a ripple in household time management. A useful and practical book for conscious cooks.

JEAN DENNEY group editor, *Mother Earth Living* and *Fermentation*

Think sourdough is just for bread? Think again! John and Jessica Moody show us how to make all your favorite grain recipes as delicious and easy-to-digest sourdough—from waffles to empanadas. Intimidated by the thought of making sourdough? Hesitate no more. *DIY Sourdough* takes you through the process step by step for foolproof recipes and lots of fun.

SALLY FALLON MORELL president, The Weston A. Price Foundation

DIY Sourdough is an easy to follow, practical guide to sourdough for the home baker. Perfect for beginners, it answers common questions that many books ignore, and focuses on simple recipes that are sure to become family favorites.

LAURIE NEVERMAN founder and blogger, Common Sense Home, author, *Never Buy Bread Again*

DIY SOURDOUGH

**JOHN AND
JESSICA MOODY**

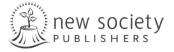

Copyright © 2020 by John Moody.
All rights reserved.
Cover design by Diane McIntosh. Cover image: ©iStock.
All images copyright John Moody unless otherwise noted.
Printed in Canada. First printing May, 2020.

Inquiries regarding requests to reprint all or part of *DIY Sourdough* should be addressed to New Society Publishers at the address below. To order directly from the publishers, please call toll-free (North America) 1-800-567-6772, or order online at www.newsociety.com

Any other inquiries can be directed by mail to:
New Society Publishers
P.O. Box 189, Gabriola Island, BC V0R 1X0, Canada
(250) 247-9737

LIBRARY AND ARCHIVES CANADA CATALOGUING IN PUBLICATION

Title: DIY sourdough : the beginner's guide to crafting starters, bread, snacks, and more / John and Jessica Moody.
Other titles: Do it yourself sourdough
Names: Moody, John (Homesteader), author. | Moody, Jessica, 1983- author.

Identifiers: Canadiana (print) 20200202197 | Canadiana (ebook) 20200202200 | ISBN 9780865719200 (softcover) | ISBN 9781550927139 (PDF) | ISBN 9781771423090 (EPUB)

Subjects: LCSH: Cooking (Sourdough) | LCSH: Sourdough bread. | LCSH: Sourdough starter. | LCGFT: Cookbooks.

Classification: LCC TX770.S66 M66 2020 | DDC 641.81/5—dc23

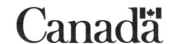

New Society Publishers' mission is to publish books that contribute in fundamental ways to building an ecologically sustainable and just society, and to do so with the least possible impact on the environment, in a manner that models this vision.

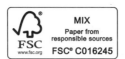 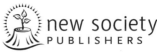

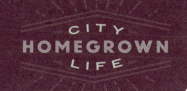

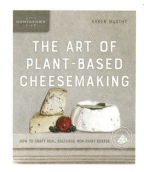

You'd like to be self-sufficient, but the space you have available is tighter than your budget. If this sounds familiar, the Homegrown City Life Series was created just for you! Our authors bring country living to the city with big ideas for small spaces. Topics include cheesemaking, fermenting, gardening, composting, and more—everything you need to create your own homegrown city life!

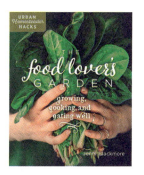

- **The Food Lover's Garden:** *Growing, Cooking and Eating Well* by Jenni Blackmore

- **The Art of Plant-Based Cheesemaking, revised & updated 2nd edition:** *How to Craft Real, Cultured, Non-Dairy Cheese* by Karen McAthy

- **Worms at Work:** *Harnessing the Awesome Power of Worms with Vermiculture and Vermicomposting* by Crystal Stevens

- **Pure Charcuterie:** *The Craft and Poetry of Curing Meats at Home* by Meredith Leigh

- DIY **Kombucha** by Andrea Potter

- DIY **Autoflowering Cannabis** by Jeff Lowenfels

- DIY **Mushroom Cultivation** by Willoughby Arevalo

- **The Elderberry Book** by John Moody

- DIY **Sourdough** by John and Jessica Moody

#Homegrowncitylife

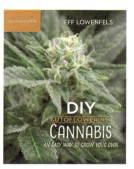

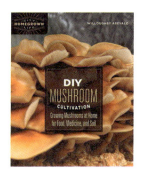

CONTENTS

ACKNOWLEDGMENTS 1

INTRODUCTION 3
How We Got into Sourdough 3
Why Sourdough? 4
Why Whole Grains? 4
Why We Recommend You Stick with Organic Grains and Flours 5
What You Need for Sourdough 6
Flour Buying Tips and Tricks 8
Grind Your Own Grains, Not As Hard As You Think 9
Grain-to-Flour Conversions 11
Home Milling Tips 12
    How Much to Mill at a Time 12
    Fineness 12
    Freshness 13

Why Spelt and Other Older
Grains for Sourdough 14

Hey, Batter Batter! The Importance
of Batter Consistency 15

1 SIMPLE SOURDOUGH BASICS 18

A Simple Sourdough Schedule 18

    Starters Take time 18

How to Create Your Own Sourdough Starter 20

Simple Step-by-Step Instructions for
Whole Grain Sourdough Starter 23

Maintaining Your Sourdough Starter 24

    Timing of Feedings and Finding
    Your Sourdough's Sweet Spot 28

    The Not-So-Uncommon Failed Sourdough Starter 28

    What to Do When You Need to
    Travel or Take a Few Days Off? 29

    The Need for a Backup Starter 30

    Waking Up Stored Starter 31

    Buying Starters 31

    Borrowing Starters 32

Common Problems that Cause
Sourdough Consternation 32

    Mold 32

    House Too Hot, House Too Cold 33

    Cross Contamination 33

    Metal and Sourdough? 34

    Too Sour 34

    Not Enough Rise 34

2 BREAKFAST 36

English Muffins 37

Hell Hath No Pastry Like My Wife's Scones 40

Pancakes and Waffles 42

Pancakes 43

Zucchini Waffles 44

French Toast 46

3 LUNCH 48

Breads 48

Irish Soda Bread/English Muffin Bread 49

Croutons 52

Crackers 54

    Rolling Crackers 54

    Scoring Crackers 54

Basic Crackers 56

    Beyond Basic Crackers 57

Artisan Spelt Bread 58

4 DINNER 64

Biscuits 65

What's the Difference Between a Biscuit, Roll, Muffin, and So Many Other Baked Goods? 67

Rolls 68

Empanadas 70

5 SNACKS AND SPECIAL TREATS 74

    Muffins 74

    Basic Muffins 75

    Blueberry Muffins 76

    Cast Iron Skillet Cinnamon Rolls 78

    Cream Cheese Frosting 81

    Cinnamon Raisin Bread 82

    Banana Bread 87

6 RESOURCES AND SUNDRY MATTERS 88

    Kitchen Equipment 88

        Cast Iron 88

        Glass 89

        Stoneware 89

        Measuring Equipment 90

        Grain Mills 91

    Online Resources 92

        Traditional Cooking School 92

        Cultures for Health 92

        Homemade Food Junkie 92

ABOUT THE AUTHORS 93

A NOTE ABOUT THE PUBLISHER 94

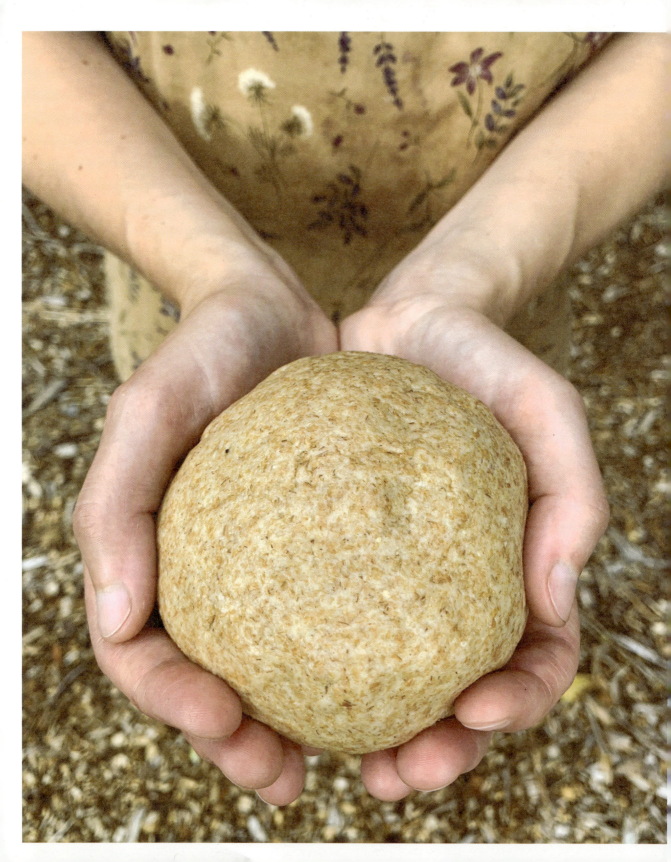

ACKNOWLEDGMENTS

WHEN I ARRIVED home from the Kansas *Mother Earth News* fair in the fall of 2018, I nonchalantly mentioned to Jessica that I had agreed to do two books over the coming eight or so months... then, I added, one was a sourdough book that we would coauthor. A bit stunned and a little uncertain, she eventually embraced the opportunity, and thus now you enjoy the fruits of our combined efforts.

Thank you to Dann Reid, who took the time right before we turned in the manuscript to give it a good read through and offered some corrections, tips, and comments to further improve it. Such is baking; sometimes you need a friend to refine your recipe!

To Ingrid and the rest of our friends at New Society, thank you again for the opportunity to help others learn skills worth having, changing the world one book at a time for the better.

To the bread of life, thank you for all the ways you have blessed and provided for our family, including the opportunity to write, speak, and teach.

To you, the reader, our appreciation. We hope you enjoy this book and the recipes as much as our family does, and hopefully even more.

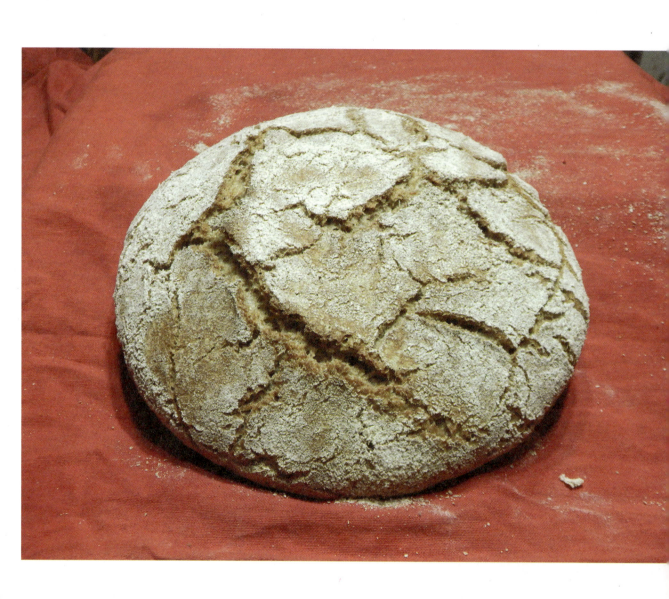

INTRODUCTION

HOW WE GOT INTO SOURDOUGH

We are a somewhat unlikely duo to write a book about sourdough. My wife hasn't eaten gluten in over a decade, though she has used traditional preparation methods for creating delightful whole grains foods for almost 15 years. My main role is taste tester, as our kids do far more of the baking than I. Some people think I can also write. So between the two of us, many thought we had something useful to add to the world of sourdough — thus our little contribution to this particular traditional art.

When we first married, we purchased a grain mill and made many different breads and other grain-based foods — pancakes, waffles, muffins, crackers, crusts — an endless array of various whole grain foods. Sue Gregg was our first influence, and then, Sally Fallon. We started to adapt our whole grain recipes to the practices and approaches used for thousands of years around the world — soaking, sprouting, sourdough — methods of harnessing nature's microbes and other natural processes to make these foods not just most nutritious but also more tasty.

Then we started having kids. Some had digestive issues that necessitated pulling them off many foods, including almost all grains for a number of years. The buying club I ran had a gifted baker join the group, who started making bread... which we eventually

"Necessity is the mother of invention."

started buying. For four years, we ate loaf after loaf of Alan's amazing sourdough breads, chicken pot pies, and other culinary creations. Until Alan moved. About six months later, I looked at Jessica one morning over breakfast saying, "Can we please eat something other than oatmeal?" Things had fallen into a rut. (She was having oatmeal anyway, since she was/is still a gluten-free gal at this time, so she really hadn't noticed any change to the routine!)

But Pinterest level sourdough production wasn't an option for our family. Five kids, some with significant learning disabilities, homeschooling, homesteading, and the "just trying to get through each day with all seven members of the family relatively whole and the house not on fire," well, we were not trying to win any awards, just hoping to create some nourishing and delicious options to keep everyone going and make lunches and other meals a bit easier.

So Jessica dived into rediscovering her inner Swedish chef and developed our family's own unique approach — simple sourdough. We don't have dozens and dozens of dishes — just a few handfuls of easy-to-make foods with consistent results. Something that often adds less than *two hours per week* to the schedule but saves us a great deal of money, while also giving us the highest-quality food for our family.

WHY SOURDOUGH?

Why would you want to eat sourdough? The answer is pretty simple—wellness. Traditional communities all across the world rarely ate whole grains without first fermenting or otherwise processing them to break down antinutrients that they contain.

Not only does sourdough decrease these antinutrients, it increases beneficial compounds in the grains, further improving their healthfulness. There is also some evidence that people who don't generally tolerate grains do tolerate sourdough quite well.

WHY WHOLE GRAINS?

Now, there are a large number of sourdough books on the market. Many, many hundreds. Some use whole grains, but often only as a small part of the recipe. Perhaps a cup of whole grain flour here or half a cup there. A few recipes comprise one-third to one-half whole grains but rarely more than that!

The preponderance of the ingredients are processed, refined flours. The problem? Refined flours not only have lost the bulk of their nutritional value and suffered oxidation of their fatty acids but also have lost their flavor. This lack of flavor and nutrition is often covered up by the addition of sugars and, in store bought breads, synthetic vitamins and minerals. If you use whole grains, especially those you mill, your baked goods will have significantly more nutrition and flavor.

But most people think using whole grains will doom their sourdough creations to a brick-like consistency, more suitable for self-defense than sustenance. And, to boot, they think that making these failures will also fill up most of their free time, a double discouragement. Sourdough doesn't have to go this way. Part of the goal of this book is to show that whole grain sourdough is both doable and delicious. While you won't get the same product as if using refined and white flours, you will create incredibly healthy and culinarily enjoyable fare for you and your friends and family.

WHY WE RECOMMEND YOU STICK WITH ORGANIC GRAINS AND FLOURS

There are many reasons to spend the premium on organic grains and flours: the problem of glyphosate applied to grains before harvest; other residual pesticides, herbicides, and fungicides; the higher nutrient content. But for sourdough makers, a recent study points to a very important consideration: the microbes that come with the grains!

> *The researchers found that the organic breads were superior in terms of specific volume, crumb structure, and crust color compared to the conventional farming system.*

What creates these incredible improvements? The wider variety and larger number of microbes found on organically grown grains!

http://microbialfoods.org/microbes-organic-flour-bread-make-better-sourdough/

WHAT IS AN ANTINUTRIENT?
Few things in nature want to be eaten — it is generally a bad survival strategy! So plants produce chemicals to try and discourage other creatures from eating them and their progeny. Many of these chemicals are *antinutrients* — they block the eater from accessing the valuable nutrients that whatever they are munching on contains. Grains contain a number of potent ones.

"Phytic acid is known as a food inhibitor which chelates micronutrient and prevents it to be bioavailable for monogastric animals, including humans, because they lack the enzyme phytase in their digestive tract. Several methods have been developed to reduce the phytic acid content in food and improve the nutritional value of cereal which becomes poor due to such antinutrients."

https://www.ncbi.nlm.nih.gov/pmc/articles/PMC4325021/

Other studies have shown that organic grains produce better starters as the grains themselves are a key component of the microbes that get your starter going. So, now you have one more reason why properly raised grains are worth the extra price!

WHAT YOU NEED FOR SOURDOUGH

Sourdough is pretty simple. Sometime in history, someone poured water on some flour and let it sit a bit too long on their counter. It began to bubble and smell. Instead of tossing this bubbling, smelly stuff, they thought of adding even more flour and water to this fermenting mixture, and behold, sourdough was born!

Basic sourdough bread is nothing more than flour, water, and salt. You will encounter one such recipe later in the book. Those three base ingredients are best thought of as the canvas on which to create a cornucopia of varying crafts. Biscuits and rolls, waffles and scones, crackers and crusts — all of these take the basic three (sometimes using a different liquid in place of water) with a few additional ingredients to make a myriad of tastes and textures.

Flour, bought or home milled: Good quality flour is very important. Milling your own is the most affordable way to create the best possible flours. Next, buying small amounts of well-sealed flours (never from open-air bulk bins!) is a great option. Whenever possible, stick with organic grains and flours.

Water, filtered: Modern standard tap water is filled with not only a wide range of contaminants but also disinfectant chemicals that kill microorganisms, like bacteria and yeast. If you can imagine, using such water to make something that relies on bacteria and yeast can significantly sabotage your efforts. So, using clean water is of utmost importance. The least expensive option is to install a filter in your house, even if it is only on your kitchen tap. The next option is to use store-bought filtered water — just make sure that it is chlorine-free! Many are not.

Salt: We prefer any number of sea salts now available on the market. We mainly use Redmond Real Salt™, but there are many good quality options for you to consider and choose among.

Cooking equipment: Here is the one rub. To make a variety of sourdough creations requires an assortment of cooking equipment. The good news? If you purchase quality pieces, your grandchildren and great-grandchildren will still be making sourdough with them long after you are laid to rest. Stoneware bread pans may seem expensive, until you realize that they will outlast their aluminum counterparts by decades — and make a superior final product. Some of our loaf pans have made hundreds of loaves and meat loaves and still are in perfect condition.

If cost is a big roadblock, you can often find used pieces at a substantial savings at yard sales, thrift stores, and the numerous places people sell unwanted items online.

Our main equipment is as follows:

- 2 stoneware bread pans (we also have 2 glass bread pans, but prefer the stone)
- 2 stoneware muffin pans
- 2 large rectangular stones (for crackers and similar creations)
- 1 cast iron muffin topper pan (for English muffins) and 1 cast iron biscuit pan (for biscuits and English muffins)
  Some of our cast iron, like our Dutch oven and skillets, get to do double duty, and are often commandeered for certain sourdough dishes, like cinnamon rolls and breads.
- A bread banneton: Although this is not required, as you can also use a bowl or strainer lined with a cloth, it is helpful.
- A waffle iron: While you don't *need* one, we find ours more than worth having on hand. This also applies to our food processor — not imperative, but definitely worth the investment in terms of time savings and labor reduction.

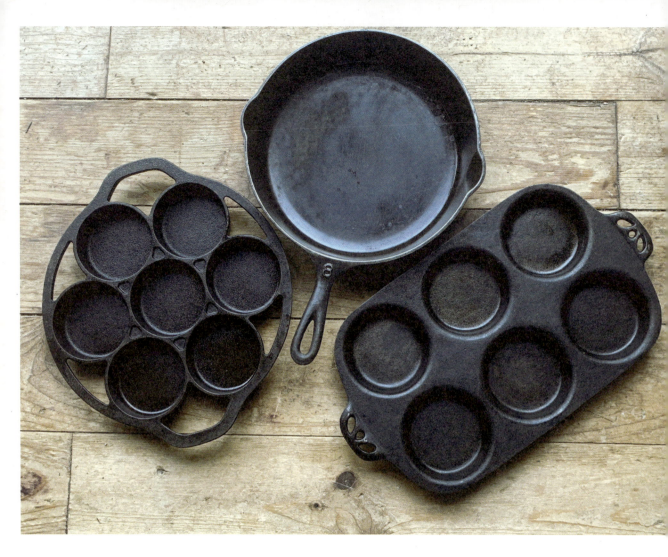

Beyond this, we use common kitchen equipment — bowls, spoons, spatulas, scissors, cutting boards, pizza cutters — nothing overly exciting or fancy, just the general pieces that make up a properly outfitted kitchen.

FLOUR BUYING TIPS AND TRICKS

If you purchase flour, there are a few ways to get the most for your money.

Never buy flour from open bins. Air + flour = oxidation. Oxidation reduces the nutritional quality of the flour along with the flavor and performance.

Resist the urge to purchase flour in bulk! Yes, it reduces the cost, but at the cost of the quality of the flour and thus all you make from it. Purchase only as much flour as you will work through in less than two to four weeks. Remember, the flour is *already* old when you get it!

Keep flour in the fridge or freezer in an airtight bag — moisture and flour *do* mix, but you don't want to let them unless it is on your terms and timing. If the flour comes in a paper bag, place that bag inside a plastic or similar bag that will not let air and moisture infiltrate.

GRIND YOUR OWN GRAINS, NOT AS HARD AS YOU THINK

The modern age has given us many gifts, some with few to no downsides. Do you really want to have to haul water and wood to make a fire to cook your food, wash your clothes, and then clean you and your kin up at the end of the day? Hot water, on demand, magically falling on my head whenever I want? What an amazing mercy.

But not all modern improvements come cost-free. Take modern breads and flours. As I sit here typing, our grain mill happily hums along in the background, taking the very shelf-stable spelt grains and cracking them open quickly and efficiently. But why go through the trouble?

First, taste. Modern processed grains lack the taste that the wide variety of traditional grains offer. From the nutty kamut to the earthy einkorn, with spelt and a dozen other grains in between, if you can grind your own grains, you can create textures and flavors that you may otherwise never get to see or experience. Modern breads do have a great deal of something — sugar, salt, and fat — to hide their lack of flavor, all three usually of low quality!

Second, nutrition. Grain berries are the storage/seed form of future plants. They are meant to keep safe all the essential nutrients and other compounds that the grain will need to create an entire new plant with hundreds of more grains. Once that seed form is broken, the protections inherent in the grain are compromised. Vitamins

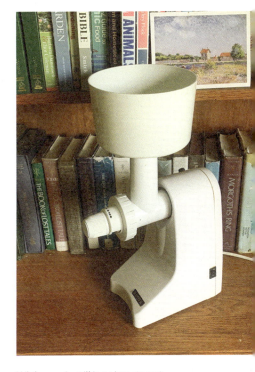

While a grain mill is an investment, it is one we and many other families have found that pays for itself in under a year.

> **IS A GRAIN MILL WORTH IT?**
>
> A grain mill is an investment, but one that pays dividends fairly quickly. Our grain mill paid for itself within the first year, and many of our friends reported similar results after they finally purchased one. A grain mill lets you buy grains in bulk, which allows you to quickly save money, compared to purchasing small amounts of flour every week or so.
>
> For example, one and a half pounds of organic spelt flour retails for around $10. That is over $6 per pound! Five pounds gets the price down to around $5 a pound. Fifty pounds of flour drops it to around $2 a pound, an incredible savings. But unless you are a bakery, the flour will go rancid far faster than you can use it.
>
> One and a half pounds of grain berries? Just over $4, or less than $3 a pound. At 10 pounds, the price is just over $2 per pound, and if you purchase 25- or 50-pound bags of the spelt berries, it drops to around $1 a pound, or half the price of the cheapest spelt flour. So you will not only save money with a grain mill but also increase the nutritional value of what you make and can experiment with all sorts of grains and other dishes that are otherwise unavailable or cost prohibitive.

begin to degrade. Fatty acids mix with oxygen and become rancid. Not only is the flavor impacted, but a once healthful food is rendered far less beneficial, if not outright problematic.

But it isn't just rancidity and oxidation that endanger milled grains. In nature, when grains become wet and conditions are right, they begin to sprout. As they do, a host of antinutrients present in the grains — which serve a key purpose in keeping the grain snug and safe until appealing growing conditions arrive — begin to break down.

Amazingly, people on every continent figured this out long ago and sought to mimic nature's ability to break down these antinutrients. But they generally didn't do it by sprouting. Instead we find a host of techniques: soaking, roasting, fermenting, sourdough.

Modern breads and flours are rarely, if ever, prepared in a way to deal with these antinutrients. Studies show we pay a heavy price for the lack of proper preparation. Some suggest that eating whole grain foods actually results in net mineral losses, along with possibly contributing to digestive and other health issues.

Our family goes through about 300 to 450 pounds of various grains (mainly spelt, oats, and buckwheat) per year. If the average savings is only $1 per pound of flour, you see how you can pay for a grain mill just in these savings. For both whole grains and larger quantities of flours, storage is as simple as a 5- or 6-gallon food-grade bucket with a Gamma Seal™ lid. These specialized lids are usually easy to purchase for under $10 and make it much easier for you to get into your buckets of grain, while also keeping insects and other problems like moisture out! $50 should let you create three or four buckets, enough to store 120 or more pounds of grain. The buckets you use to store grains and flours must be kept in a cool, relatively dry, dark place.

A number of grains, if you purchase a 50-pound bag, won't fit in a 5-gallon bucket. In such situations, we just use a smaller sealed container for the excess and work through that first.

The best news? If you have a KitchenAid or similar appliance, milling your own grains is just a matter of getting an appropriate attachment. While a stand-alone grain mill is more expensive, a good one will last you many years. Ours is over a decade old, and other than replacing the milling head for under $30 and the fuse a few times for a dollar or two, it has given us no issues. That pencils out to about $30 per year to create hundreds of English muffins and loaves of breads, boxes and boxes of crackers, waffles, muffins, and so much else. You are looking at less than 10 cents a day to make your own nutritious, traditional foods.

GRAIN-TO-FLOUR CONVERSIONS

A cup (which is a measurement of volume) of grain berries and a cup of flour are not the same! Flour contains more air space and, thus, is less dense. So knowing generally how to get from whole grain berries to flour is important and the below table serves as a good general guide.

General grain-to-flour conversions

GRAIN BERRIES	FLOUR
½ cup	¾ cup
⅔ cup	1 cup
1 cup	1½ cups
1⅓ cups	2 cups
1½ cups	2¼ cups
1⅔ cups	2½ cups
2 cups	3 cups
2½ cups	3¾ cups
3 cups	4½ cups
3½ cups	5¼ cups
4 cups	6 cups
¾ cup of spelt berries = 1 cup spelt flour	
⅔ cup of wheat berries = 1 cup of wheat flour	

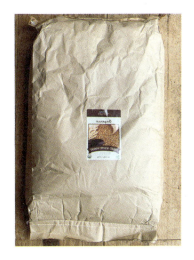

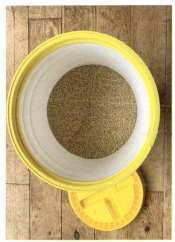

Keeping grains around in their bags is an invitation for problems, from small pests like bugs to larger ones like mice. For about $10, you can create a safe, secure, and easily accessible storage method using a bucket and a Gamma Seal lid.

HOME MILLING TIPS

How Much to Mill at a Time

Not only is a cup of whole grains not equal to a cup of flour, but different grains yield slightly different amounts of flour, and each recipe needs adjusted some for the particular grain you choose to use.

One reason some bakers incorporate a small amount of rye into their baking is because it naturally extends the shelf life.

With einkorn, don't be tempted to increase the amount of flour instead of reducing the amount of liquid, as this doesn't work!

Since most grain mills are slow, while they work is a perfect time to get other tasks done. It is not uncommon, since we mill in the afternoon or early evening, to tidy up the kitchen or attend to other close at hand work while making fresh flour. Also note, kids around six to eight and older are perfect helpers to assist with the milling. This way it doesn't really add much extra time to your routine.

Generally speaking, you want to mill a bit more flour than the recipe calls for, since you may need extra for kneading or other purposes. Any that you don't use can be fed to your starter over the next few days, so nothing will go to waste.

Fineness

Sometimes, either because of a recipe's requirements or because of your mill, your flour won't come out fine enough, adversely affecting your final creation. In such situations, you should run your grains through *twice*. The key is to mill them moderately coarse on the first run through, and then at the finest setting the second time. If you mill them too fine the first time, the flour generally won't happily go through the mill a second. So, if you need to grind twice to get a finer flour, don't set the mill to the finest setting first run!

COMMON FLOUR-TO-FLOUR CONVERSIONS

If a recipe requires 1 cup of whole wheat flour, it will use about:

- 1¼ cups spelt flour or
- ⅞ cup kamut flour or
- 1 cup einkorn flour, but you will generally need to reduce the liquid portion of the recipe by 15–30%

For rye, most recipes replace anywhere from 5 to 50 percent of the flour with rye flour.

CHOOSING A GRAIN MILL

Some earlier models of grain mills had one rather unfortunate design flaw: they became quite hot when milling, which damaged both the flavor and nutritional value of the grains. While it seems more recent models no longer suffer from this design defect, when selecting among milling options, make sure to inquire about this issue — How does the mill handle prolonged milling, and does it become unsuitably hot during the process?

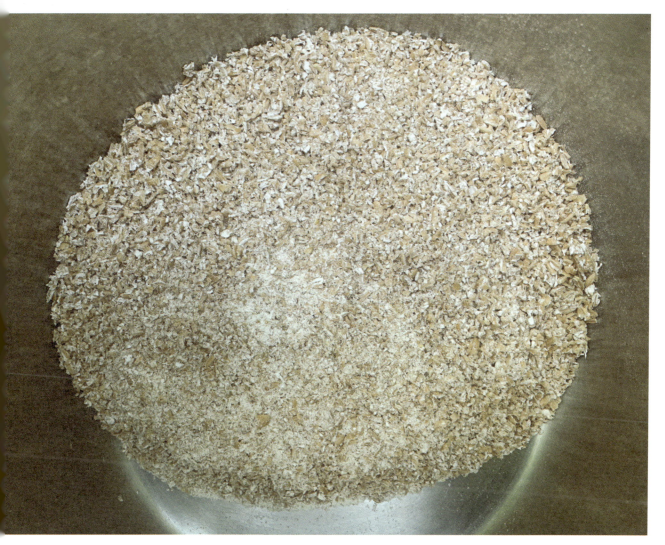

Some grain mills cannot create fine flour on the first run. For such mills, grind the grains coarsely to start and then a second time to achieve a finer finished flour.

Freshness

Sometimes, you miscalculate and end up with a little extra flour. Or, you know you are about to have a busy week. So, instead of trying to make flour every day to feed your starter, you mill just twice a week to simplify your schedule. The latter is what we do, milling only on the days we bake.

If you end up with some leftover flour, or need to mill ahead some for your starter, here is how to keep the flour fresh:

- Immediately after milling, place the flour into a small, airtight container or bag. Press out any excess air.
- Place the container in your fridge or freezer.
- Ideally, use the flour within 3 to 4 days of milling.

WHY SPELT AND OTHER OLDER GRAINS FOR SOURDOUGH

While we primarily use spelt, most of the recipes in the book have proportions for both spelt and wheat. But why do we use spelt? There are a number of reasons, the first being taste and texture. If you have never tried some of the many traditional grains — spelt, einkorn, kamut — you are missing out! Each of these grains has a unique flavor that can enhance or help create amazing dishes that most people will never get to enjoy.

The second reason we use spelt, and sometimes kamut or einkorn, is for our health. Modern wheats are highly hybridized, that is, crossed with other related species to create new strains. While this was beneficial in some ways — especially for increasing yields or decreasing difficulty in harvesting done by heavy equipment — it also had numerous drawbacks. These included decreased resistance to pests and disease, much lower nutritional density, and altered protein profiles that a number of doctors and researchers now link to problematic health conditions. Most modern grains contain significantly less protein and nutrients than their older counterparts like spelt and kamut.

Many traditional grains, when prepared in traditional ways, including sourdough, are often well tolerated, if not outright health promoting, for those who otherwise have significant problems consuming products containing modern wheat. Also, many of these grains are grown without the harsh herbicides and pesticides used on modern wheat cultivars.

One thing to note, especially with spelt, but also true for einkorn and to some degree kamut, is that the protein is more fragile than that found in modern wheats. Thus, over-kneading or over-working batters and doughs can cause deleterious results.

HEY, BATTER BATTER!
THE IMPORTANCE OF BATTER CONSISTENCY

Since each grain has a unique composition, while you can substitute almost any grain, it is rarely a perfect one-to-one substitution. For instance, our main grain — spelt — requires more flour than most standard wheats. A recipe that uses 2 cups of wheat flour will often take close to 2½ of spelt. So, for many recipes, we have provided measurements for both spelt and hard red wheat.

Also, how thick or thin you keep your starter can make a few spoonfuls difference to a recipe's final flour amounts. So, when prepping a recipe, I also take our starter's current state into consideration. We generally aim for a firm but slightly sticky dough.

I consider not only the number of cups a recipe calls for but also the thickness/consistency and moistness of the dough or batter. Keep in mind that often a dough will become a bit drier/less sticky overnight so you can leave it a tad wetter than you normally would so as not to over-flour. On the other hand, batters tend to break down as the sourdough works its magic and become slightly thinner by morning. As with any baking or cooking, there is an element of science mixed with art and experience that you will develop a feel for over time.

Besides the type of flour you use, other variables can affect the amount of flour needed to achieve the correct consistency, including the thickness of the starter (sometimes it may be thicker or thinner than usual) and the level of moisture in the flour. The moisture level can vary depending on how old the grain or flour is, how it is stored, and the humidity, which varies substantially in some places throughout the year (like our kitchen!).

These are all good reasons to become adept at determining proper dough and batter texture for the various recipes, and we have included pictures of the batters and doughs to help you. Typically, dough recipes will have more variance in flour amounts, whereas batter recipes will be consistent.

SIMPLE SOURDOUGH BASICS

A SIMPLE SOURDOUGH SCHEDULE

What is the most important part of sourdough success? Having a sourdough schedule that you can stick with. And what kind of schedule is the easiest to stick with? A simple one! So below we will go over our simple approach to keeping the crew in sourdough.

Think of sourdough as a pet — it has daily and weekly needs. If you meet those needs, it will reward you. If you don't, it won't. The problem is many people's sourdough falls into neglect. They can't figure out a schedule to manage it that doesn't at the same time drive them mad. Here is our simplified sourdough schedule.

Note, since we mill only once or twice a week, we mill enough flour to cover all the other days of feeding at the same time. Milling for feeding is done on the day before bake days, since the mill is already out. The extra flour is stored in the fridge or freezer. Since you are only adding a few spoonfuls to your starter at a time, if you are worried that the cold might negatively affect it, scoop it out about 15 minutes before you feed it. We have not had any issues going straight from freezer to feeding.

Starters Take Time

Making your own sourdough starter is not hard, but it does take time. After 3 weeks, your starter will be ready to make some tasty

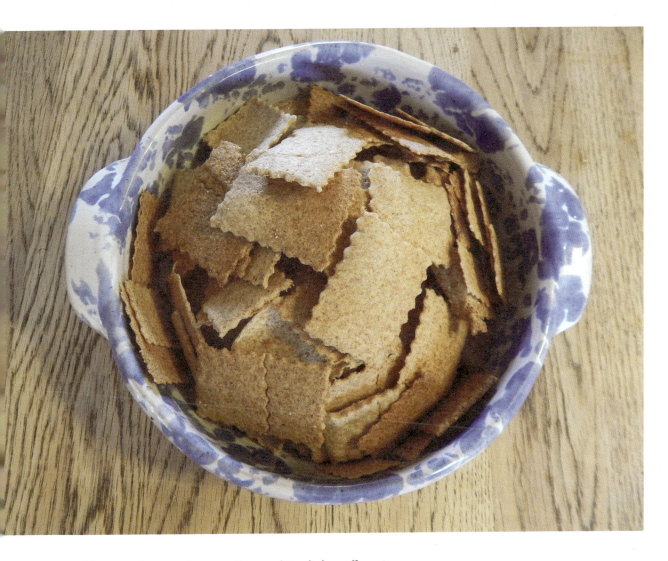

treats like pancakes, crackers, muffins, and English muffins. Over the next several months, the starter will continue to mature, and its rising power will increase quite a bit. At first, the baked goods you make using your new starter may taste fairly sour. Over time, as your starter matures, this sour taste mellows. Using recipes that include baking soda with a new starter can help you get through those first weeks and months until your starter's taste has mellowed and its leavening power optimizes.

Not only does sourdough take time but you also must be consistent. This goes both for when making your starter and when

> **BABIES AND BACKUP STARTER**
>
> Early one morning, I heard a shriek in the kitchen. Not quite a scream, but the noise of immense sadness emanating from Jessica. I dashed out of my office to ask what had happened and saw her hunched over a glass jar — okay, not any glass jar, but her just starting to get to that mature, established sourdough starter stage glass jar. It also was the jar that our one-and-a-half-year-old had just poured a large amount of homemade salad dressing into… ruining the starter. Four months of work, almost entirely ruined in under 40 seconds. Jess was able to — after ten or so minutes of work — salvage a few spoonfuls of uncontaminated starter culture. It was just enough, but it was a close call we decided was never worth repeating.
>
> It was a reminder that, every so often, you should make sure you back up your starter.

maintaining the starter's strength and health over time. We feed the starter twice a day; during the hottest times of the year, we will switch to three times a day.

This only takes a minute or so per day but helps protect the starter from mold growth and other problems. If you forget one day, it is no big deal. But if you neglect to work quick starter care into your routine, you will have a much harder time making consistent, successful sourdough.

HOW TO CREATE YOUR OWN SOURDOUGH STARTER

It doesn't take great skill or expense to create your own fantastic sourdough starter. What does it take? Time and consistent, though not time-consuming, care on your part. Some people suggest creating your starter using particular grains, such as rye, but we used spelt and had no issues achieving success.

Before my wife started her sourdough culture, she read numerous resources, and was greatly helped by the tips given at the Traditional Cooking School. Our process is very similar to the one they recommend.

Start with a clean pint glass jar or a small bowl. Clear glass is particularly useful as it allows you to see activity in your new starter from the sides in addition to the surface. In the jar, combine ¼ cup of whole spelt or whole wheat flour and just under ¼ cup of water (ends up being just over ⅜ cup, if you're measuring). Some people like to measure by weight rather than volume. That takes more time and precision than we feel is necessary at this stage, but if you would like to do that, measure an equal amount (by weight) of flour and water; about 30 grams of each would be good for creating a new starter.

Mix together thoroughly, scrape down the sides, and loosely cover with a clean cloth. We like to use a cloth napkin for this purpose, held in place by a rubber band if needed. Allow to sit for 12 hours in a warm spot out of direct sunlight.

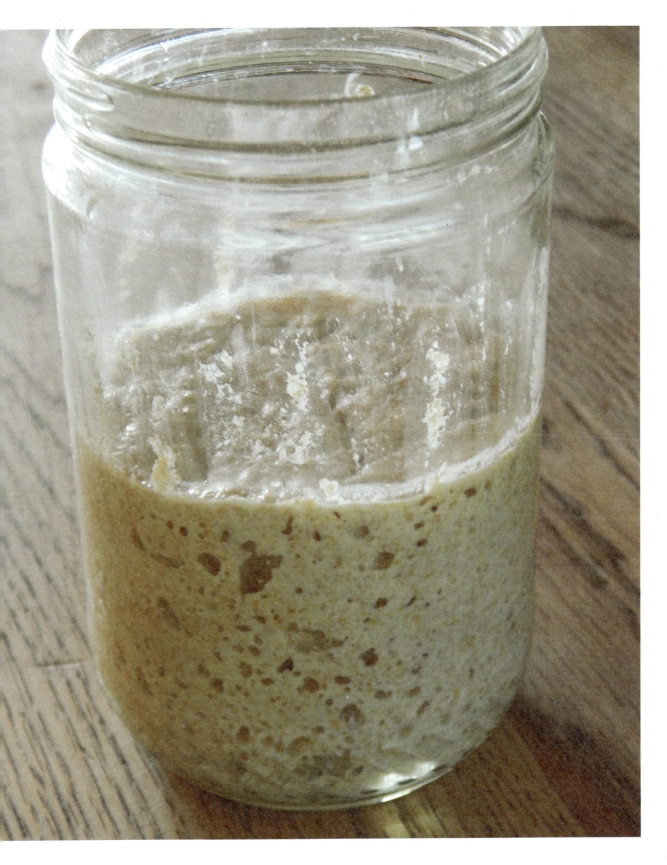

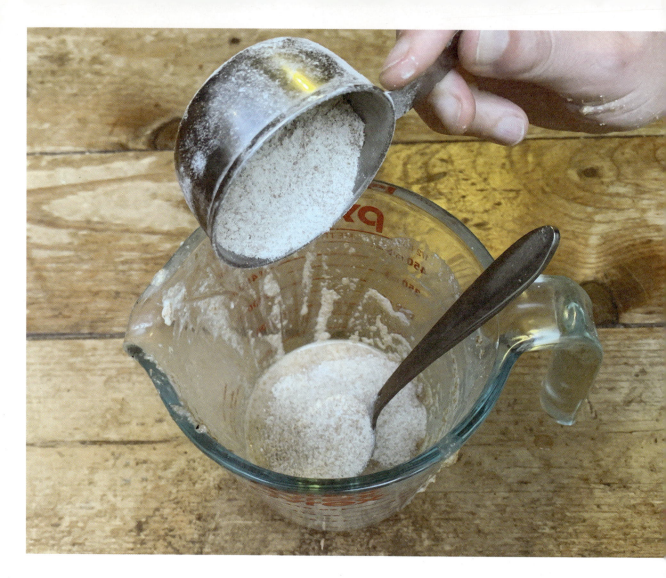

After approximately 12 hours, remove half of the mixture and discard; chickens or pigs, compost piles, or worm bins will all appreciate this healthy addition to their regular diet.

Now add another ¼ cup of flour and just under ¼ cup of water. Mix together thoroughly, scrape down the sides, cover, and let sit for another 12 hours.

This is the basic routine for getting your starter going. Every 12 or so hours, remove half of the mixture, add ¼ cup flour and just under ¼ cup water, stir well, scrape down sides, cover with a cloth, allow to sit 12 hours, and then repeat. Between days 4 and 7, you should start to see bubbles and sniff a slightly sour smell — the beginnings of your starter's soon to be rich and diverse microbial mix!

If you are using wheat flour, once your starter is active, it will double in the jar and large air holes will be visible through the sides. Spelt, and perhaps other traditional grains, does not increase in size so noticeably, but you will see lots of tiny bubbles both on the sides and on top. This is most likely due to the lower gluten content and different protein profiles among the various grains.

After about 3 weeks, your starter is ready to use. At this point, you can also reduce the twice-daily feedings to 1 tablespoon of flour and just less than 1 tablespoon of water. Continue to scrape the sides and keep covered with a cloth.

Below are step-by-step instructions for making your own starter from scratch.

SIMPLE STEP-BY-STEP INSTRUCTIONS FOR WHOLE GRAIN SOURDOUGH STARTER

Day 1 morning: Combine ¼ cup whole grain flour and ⅜ cup filtered water in a clean pint jar. Stir well, scrape down sides, cover loosely with a cloth.

Day 1 evening: Remove half of your starter and add ¼ cup whole grain flour and ⅜ cup filtered water. Stir well, scrape down sides, cover loosely with a cloth.

Day 2 morning: Remove half of your starter and add ¼ cup whole grain flour and ⅜ cup filtered water. Stir well, scrape down sides, cover loosely with a cloth.

Day 2 evening: Remove half of your starter and add ¼ cup whole grain flour and ⅜ cup filtered water. Stir well, scrape down sides, cover loosely with a cloth.

Day 3 morning: Remove half of your starter and add ¼ cup whole grain flour and ⅜ cup filtered water. Stir well, scrape down sides, cover loosely with a cloth.

Day 3 evening: Remove half of your starter and add ¼ cup whole grain flour and ⅜ cup filtered water. Stir well, scrape down sides, cover loosely with a cloth.

By this time, you should start to see bubbles forming on the sides and top of your starter. This lets you know you are on the right track. Over time, you will see more activity as the starter becomes stronger. Continue to remove ½ of your starter and feed it with ¼ cup whole grain flour and ⅜ cup filtered water twice a day for 3 weeks. After 3 weeks, your starter is ready to use but may not be strong enough for making breads just yet. Continue to feed twice a day, but you no longer need to discard half of the starter. So that I don't have way more starter on hand than I need at this point, I switch to adding just 1 tablespoon of flour and 1 scant tablespoon of water at each feeding.

Now it's time to move from making a starter to maintaining it.

MAINTAINING YOUR SOURDOUGH STARTER

Congratulations! Your starter is officially no longer a newborn! But it still has a number of months to go before it is a mature sourdough starter. As mentioned above, you can now reduce the amount of water and flour fed to your sourdough twice daily. You also no longer need to discard a portion of the starter during these during these feedings. But how much sourdough starter should you keep on hand?

I like to keep about ⅛ to ½ a cup of starter in my main jar at a time. Many recipes require more starter than I keep on hand. For instance, the English muffin recipe requires ½ cup of starter, which I will need the night before I plan to make them. So, the morning before, I will feed the starter enough flour and water to make ½ cup plus ⅛ to ½ cup extra. Basically, feed enough to get the amount for the recipe along with sufficient leftover starter.

WHAT ABOUT STARTERS THAT USE ALL PURPOSE OR BREAD FLOUR?

As we have already explained, we typically use whole grains in our sourdough starter, but what if you have or are given a starter that is made with all purpose or bread flour? The great thing is you can use it for all the recipes in this book. If you want, you can easily convert an all purpose flour starter to a whole grain one simply by feeding it a whole grain flour of your choice. Whole wheat, spelt, einkorn, and rye all work great in our recipes. You can also continue to feed it with all purpose or bread flour. Starters that don't use whole grains are quite different in consistency, but they will still work well — in fact, some people who make whole grain sourdough breads maintain their starters with all purpose flour.

You may wonder, why keep so little starter on hand? Since you are feeding it twice daily your starter will grow in size every day until you remove some for baking. Also, by keeping a smaller amount on hand, it means that, two feedings before we bake, the starter requires a larger feeding. In our experience, this larger feeding — usually doubling the amount in the jar — produces better results with our sourdough creations because it makes the starter quite vigorous and active.

Just to make sure it is clear, this oversized feeding takes place a full 24 hours before baking. So if we plan to make bread Saturday morning, on Friday morning the starter will get a larger feeding. Friday night, we will use the starter to make the dough that will then be baked Saturday morning. If we are going to make crackers Monday afternoon, then on Sunday afternoon or evening, we will make sure the starter is fed so that Monday morning, when we mix the dough, we have the right amount for the recipe and leftover starter.

Here are a few sample sourdough schedules to give you an idea how you can easily incorporate making sourdough a few times a week into your schedule.

A SIMPLE GUIDE TO GRAINS		
	PRICE PER POUND	NOTES
Soft White Wheat	$0.60	Generally used for pastries.
Hard White Wheat	$0.60	Whole grain, but tends to have a lighter texture.
Hard Red Wheat	$0.60	Typical bread grain used by many home bakers.
Emmer (Farro)	$1.40	Similar flavor and texture to spelt.
Rye	$0.70	Strong flavor, often used in small amounts with other grains.
Spelt	$1.10	Older grain, excellent flavor.
Kamut	$1.30	Nutty flavor, naturally lower in gluten.
Einkorn	$2.50	Considered an "ancient grain," only non-hybridized strain commercially available.

TWO RECIPE EXAMPLE SOURDOUGH SCHEDULE - EXAMPLE 1		
Monday	Morning	Feed starter to make 1¼ cups.
	Evening	Remove 1 cup starter. Prepare a double of English Muffin dough (page 26).
		Feed starter 1 tablespoon flour and scant 1 tablespoon water.
Tuesday	Morning	Feed starter. Bake English Muffins.
	Evening	Feed starter.
Wednesday	Morning	Feed starter.
	Evening	Feed starter.
Thursday	Morning	Feed starter.
	Evening	Feed starter.
Friday	Morning	Feed starter.
	Evening	Feed starter to make 2¾ cups.
Saturday	Morning	Remove 2½ cups starter. Make Waffles or Pancakes (page 42).
		Feed starter.
	Evening	Feed starter.
Sunday	Morning	Feed starter.
	Evening	Feed starter.

THREE RECIPE SOURDOUGH SCHEDULE - EXAMPLE 1		
Monday	Morning	Feed starter 1 tablespoon flour and scant 1 tablespoon water.
	Evening	Feed starter to make 1¼ cups.
Tuesday	Morning	Remove 1 cup starter. Make Cracker dough (Page 56).
		Feed starter.
	Afternoon	Bake Crackers.
	Evening	Feed starter.
Wednesday	Morning	Feed starter to make 1 cup.
	Evening	Remove ¾ cup of starter. Mix up Muffins (page 75).
Thursday	Morning	Bake Muffins.
		Feed starter.
	Evening	Feed starter.
Friday	Morning	Feed starter to make ½ cup.
	Afternoon	Remove ¼ cup starter. Make Artisan Bread dough (page 58).
	Evening	Feed starter and follow Artisan Bread recipe (refrigerate dough).
Saturday	Morning	Feed starter and follow Artisan Bread recipe.
	Afternoon	Bake Artisan Bread.
	Evening	Feed starter.
Sunday	Morning	Feed starter.
	Evening	Feed starter.

TWO RECIPE SOURDOUGH SCHEDULE - EXAMPLE 2		
Monday	Morning	Feed starter 1 tablespoon flour and scant 1 tablespoon water.
	Evening	Feed starter.
Tuesday	Morning	Feed Starter. Bake English Muffins.
	Evening	Remove ¾ cup of starter. Prepare Irish Soda Bread dough (page 49).
		Feed starter.
Wednesday	Morning	Feed starter. Make Irish Soda Bread.
	Evening	Feed starter.
Thursday	Morning	Feed starter.
	Evening	Feed starter.
Friday	Morning	Feed starter to make 1¾ cups.
	Evening	Remove 1½ cups starter and prepare a double of Empanada crust (page 72).
		Feed Starter. Prepare Empanada filling (page 70).
Saturday	Morning	Feed starter.
		Prepare and bake Empanadas.
	Evening	Feed starter.
Sunday	Morning	Feed starter.
	Evening	Feed starter.

THREE RECIPE SOURDOUGH STARTER - EXAMPLE 2		
Monday	Morning	Feed starter 1 tablespoon flour and scant 1 tablespoon water.
	Evening	Feed starter.
Tuesday	Morning	Feed starter to make ¾ cup.
	Evening	Prepare Scone dough (Page 40).
		Feed starter.
Wednesday	Morning	Feed starter to make ¾ cup. Bake Scones.
	Evening	Feed starter.
Thursday	Morning	Feed starter to ¾ cup.
	Evening	Prepare Banana Bread batter (page 87).
	Evening	Feed starter.
Friday	Morning	Bake Banana Bread.
	Evening	Feed starter.
Saturday	Morning	Feed starter to make ¾ cup.
	Evening	Prepare Cinnamon Roll dough (page 78).
Sunday	Morning	Feed starter.
		Bake Cinnamon Rolls.
	Evening	Feed starter.

WHY WATER IS SO IMPORTANT

Most people are on city or municipal water, which contains both chlorine and fluoride. These chemicals are problematic for home food preservation and fermentation, as both act as microbe murderers. They can significantly weaken if not outrightly undo your efforts.

So, if you are on treated water, you will either want to install some type of filtration, especially to remove the chlorine and chlorine by-products or need to purchase distilled or similar water that is free of these chemicals that will adversely affect your attempts at sourdough.

Timing of Feedings and Finding Your Sourdough's Sweet Spot

The goal with your starter is to give it more food, right when it is at the peak of its activity. But how can you tell that your starter is ready? If you look carefully at your starter, instead of the top surface sitting flat, it will have a slightly domed shape from the strength of the fermentation taking place. This, along with the presence of air bubbles all over the starter (which is one reason we prefer a glass container, as it allows you to see this activity beyond just the surface) are the signs that tell you it is ready for another feeding.

If there are bubbles, but the top has fallen back down or flattened out, you may have waited too long. As a general rule, we feed the starter in the morning and evening, approximately (but not slavishly) 12 hours apart. During the summer, particularly on very hot days when our house will often approach the high 70s, these clues let us notice that sometimes our starter benefits from an additional afternoon feeding.

The Not-So-Uncommon Failed Sourdough Starter

Our first attempt at sourdough came over a decade ago. After following some directions with extreme diligence for over a week to get our first starter going, Jessica made our first loaf of sourdough bread. The cookbook said the starter would be ready for bread making in just 7 days. The bread wasn't bad... if you enjoy eating a cross between completely sweetless Sour Patch Kids mixed with overwatered concrete. Needless to say, between our early failures and adding two kids to our crew in a little over two years, we dropped sourdough.

This is not an uncommon mistake (nor uncommon advice in a number of books!); many new sourdough makers become discouraged by their early only semi-edible results and toss their starter and sourdough aspirations in the compost pile or trash can.

A good starter needs around 3 to 4 months to achieve an acceptable, balanced flavor and sufficient strength to create good rise. It takes about 6 to 8 months to reach a solid, mature state. This is one reason that if you can get sourdough starter from an experienced maker, you will save yourself many months.

In the meantime, if you start your starter from scratch, you don't have to take care of your little sourdough baby for 3 months with no immediate payoff. Instead, after about 3 weeks — once you are getting good, consistent bubbly action and other signs of sourdough success — you can start with some of the simple recipes and options, especially crackers, pancakes and waffles, and English muffins. If you find these are a bit too tangy at first, slightly increase the amount of baking soda. Remember, with additional time, your starter will mellow and achieve an excellent flavor. Think of it like parenting: the challenging preteen and teen years eventually give way to the more mellow 20s if you persevere!

What to Do When You Need to Travel or Take a Few Days Off?

Life happens. Even with a great schedule, sometimes you won't get to your sourdough, or you will need to be away from home for a few days or longer. Kids end up in the ER. Cars break down. Potatoes need planting. Work calls you in for an extra shift. The stomach bug invades your family.

How can you avoid undoing all your hard work to get a great starter? Feed your sourdough and tuck it in the fridge for a few days, or even a week. It will be fine. When you get back to it, note that it may need a few days to wake up and regather its strength. But otherwise, your starter should still be its former excellent self.

Old-timers used to travel with their sourdough, but we think that the TSA and other agencies may frown upon such sourdough smuggling. Though, seriously, if you are away for an extended time, do not hesitate to find a way to take your DLS (dear little starter) with you. Maybe classify it as an "emotional support starter"?

Also, life with all its unexpected lessons is a good reason why sharing starters is such a great idea. When we began making kombucha many years ago, we shared scobies with dozens of people.

After a horrible brewing debacle that killed our scoby and a large (60-plus-gallon) batch of kombucha, we had to start over! But instead of having to order starter in or create one from scratch, we hunted down some of the many offspring of our scoby now spread far and wide among our friends and community, who were more than happy to return some of what we gave to them months, or sometimes years, before. We are now building up progeny of our sourdough starter throughout our area, knowing that one day something may happen to ours that others will help us remedy. It also isn't a bad idea to have your own backup starter. So let's talk about how.

The Need for a Backup Starter

It is important, as part of your schedule, to ensure you create a backup sourdough culture, for when things go wrong. Things like one of your kids dropping the starter and its container shattering into a million pieces, embedding countless shards of glass in your sourdough.

There are three ways to create a backup: freezer, fridge, and dehydrator. For the first method, freeze about ½ to 1 cup of your starter, right *after* feeding. You should rotate your frozen backup starter every 4 to 6 months. The second method is placing a backup in your refrigerator right *after* feeding. Feed the starter, and place about ½ to 1 cup in the coldest part of your fridge. Feed it once a week if possible. As with the freezer method, we suggest rotating it every 4 to 6 months. If you neglect to feed it weekly, you may want to rotate it sooner.

With the third method, take 1 cup of starter and spread it thinly on a dehydrator sheet. Dehydrate until it is a cracker-like consistency, and place it into an airtight bag. Put it back into your fridge or freezer.

Jessica prefers having at least two methods of backup: fridge and freezer. Given the exciting times our two-year-old is currently creating for the family, I am almost tempted to keep a few spare starters in every room of the house!

Waking Up Stored Starter

If you need to use a backup starter that is frozen or refrigerated, it will require a few days to "wake up" before it will be ready to use. For frozen starters, transfer them to the fridge and thaw 2 or so days. Once thawed, or when working with a refrigerated starter, allow it to come to room temperature. After pouring off any excess liquid sitting on top of the stored starter, scoop 4 tablespoons or so of it into a clean container. Feed it by adding 1 tablespoon of flour and just less than 1 tablespoon of water, mixing it all together well.

Allow it to sit for 12 hours and feed again. Resume the normal twice-daily feeding schedule. In 2 to 4 days, you should see a vibrant sourdough starter back in action. If, after 4 to 5 days, you are not seeing bubbles and other signs of sourdough life, or if mold or other problems take place, compost the starter and use your other backup or one you shared with a friend! This is unusual in our experience, but can happen.

Note that making your own starter isn't the only option on the table. Many places have people or groups that love to share starters. A number of companies and businesses now also sell starters. So let's briefly talk about these options.

Buying Starters

Many local artisan businesses now sell starters, and many larger companies, such as Cultures for Health, sell them nationally and internationally. You can now find starters in many specialty stores! While working on this book, we had the pleasure of trying out two starters from Cultures for Health! They are easy to activate, and once that's done, you are ready to go with a healthy, active starter in only one week! Cultures for Health has offered a 20% discount to our readers, good for one use on any sourdough cultures or supplies. (Just use the code DIYSD20.)

Borrowing Starters

Another great way to get sourdough going is to borrow starter from someone in your area. While buying starters isn't a bad option, shipping living things — such as a sourdough starter — is dicey business. Temperature, air, and so much else can weaken or outright kill a starter during shipment. With a local person, you run into none of these issues, and often can just barter, trade, or get pro bono. Don't worry if you are not given a whole grain starter. It can easily be converted simply by feeding it with your choice of whole grain flour. In my experience, it takes 3 or 4 days to begin adjusting to a different type of flour, but after that, you should be able to bake with it without issue.

COMMON PROBLEMS THAT CAUSE SOURDOUGH CONSTERNATION

Mold

Our dear daughter has created this problem by feeding the starter, and then not properly stirring and then scraping down the sides of the glass jar. The fresh sticky mixture, thinly spread up toward the top, is an inviting target for mold. My more conscientious wife has never had this issue, as after feeding, she takes a moment to scrape the sides of the jar. Also, every time she bakes with the starter (generally twice a week), she switches to a new clean jar.

If you neglect your starter, you may also run into mold. You can, if the mold is not too well established and over-running the starter, remove any liquid, and then take a clean tablespoon of starter from the bottom of the starter mixture — the mold usually forms on the top or on the sides of the jar. Feed this as normal, and give it 4 or so days to be brought back to health.

House Too Hot, House Too Cold

A sourdough starter prefers a temperature around 72° to 74°F.

For us, the house (unless the HVAC breaks) is rarely too hot, save in late July through late August. If your house is too hot, try keeping your starter in the coolest spot possible — this may be an interior closet or similar location. You may also need to feed it 3 instead of 2 times per day.

If your house is too cold, which is generally the more common conundrum, you should keep your starter in the warmest place possible, such as on top of your fridge (which is generally a few degrees warmer than elsewhere in your home) or on your stovetop.

If your house is really cold, then a heat mat may be the best option. These are inexpensive and have a low energy cost as well, especially compared to increasing the temperature of your entire home just for the sake of your sourdough. If you live farther north, or like to keep your house on the cooler side, this is a must for successful sourdough.

Starters should not be stored in direct sunlight! Sunlight is a natural antimicrobial — it kills bacteria and yeast, so it is not very compatible with the microorganisms that make sourdough success.

Cross Contamination

It's a bacteria-eat-bacteria world out there! If you do a number of other ferments, it is important to keep them somewhat separated. So, if you are a kombucha brewer, don't keep your sourdough starter right next to your kombucha tank. Making sauerkraut or pickles? They should sit on a different counter space than your sourdough. Same goes for tools and utensils. Any that are used across ferments need to be thoroughly washed after use.

Stainless steel is best, as wooden utensils can, even after a good washing with soap and water, contain a great deal of (good) microorganisms that can make their way into your other ferments. Since different ferments do best with slightly to very different mixes of microbes, cross contamination can be a small to catastrophic issue in your kitchen. Best to avoid it all together and practice good personal and kitchen hygiene!

Metal and Sourdough?

Some people say you should never use metal kitchenware — spoons and other such implements — with your sourdough. You can use a dedicated wooden spoon if you want to, but we have always used our standard kitchen silverware (stainless steel) and other stainless steel kitchen tools. We have never, ever, ever had an issue. They are also vastly easier to clean and work with compared to wooden tools.

Too Sour

Your starter may need a few more months to mature. Or, for a mature starter, you may need to increase how often you are feeding it— remembering to remove some of the old sour starter before feeding.

Not Enough Rise

This again is sometimes because a starter is either immature and needs a few more months to gather its strength or because of inconsistent feeding. House temperature (too cool or too warm) can also cause this issue. If it gets rather hot in the summer (high 70s and above), you may need to feed your starter three times a day, since the increased temperatures will speed up its fermentation.

Address the underlying issues, and that should go a long way toward improving your starter's performance. You can also create "super starter," which we talk about in chapter 3, when you need max rising power.

EXCESS STARTER

What to do if you end up with too much starter? Perhaps you missed making anything for a week or so but kept feeding... and feeding... and feeding your sourdough faithfully, only for it to threaten to take over your entire kitchen!

You can use some of it to create backup starters, tossing it into a jar to keep in the fridge. But at some point, someone may begin to question your sanity if you start to run out of fridge space because of so many sourdough starters squirreled away. (I haven't done this to Jessica... yet... but we are getting close, especially now that she wants to start a third different sourdough starter!) Pancakes and waffles are a great way to dispose of excess starter; the recipes use a large amount. If you have animals, in particular, chickens or pigs, excess sourdough starter is an excellent addition to their diet; they will thrive from all the beneficial bacteria and yeast that your starter shares.

Excess starter is also fine to add to your compost or worm compost. With worm compost, only add in small amounts, such as a ½ cup or so at a time, so that it doesn't cause problems or attract pests.

Don't forget that people are often searching for sourdough starter, so don't be afraid to ask around to see if anyone in your area is in need.

BREAKFAST

THERE ARE MANY foods I remember from my childhood. Jessica is always amazed at the rich culinary roots that my native Northeast Ohio instilled in me, and the number of strange foods that she had never heard of until we wed. Wedding soup and pizzelles. Perogies and potato boats. English muffin bread — a breakfast treat that my mom would have to hide from me and my siblings, lest the loaves last not even a day!

So it is no surprise that our foray into sourdough began with breakfast woes, and one of the first foods Jessica mastered was an English muffin. Which, like my mom, she now has to hide (or make in triple and quadruple batches) lest none last past the first day.

ENGLISH MUFFINS

This is the recipe we use most in the entire book. These get triple duty — breakfast, lunch, and dinner: sausage or Canadian bacon and egg English muffins, sandwiches (we find these are the easiest bread option for sandwich making, especially on school days!), and as a side with dinners when we need to add some bulk to a meal.

You will need one or two special trays to make these, either a cast iron or stoneware muffin topper pan or a biscuit pan. Why cast iron or stoneware? They do the best job holding and transferring heat, giving the muffins a nice crisp exterior while ensuring the interior is fully cooked.

1. The night before, combine starter, milk, and honey, mixing thoroughly. Add flour until a soft dough forms. You want it to still be somewhat sticky, adding just enough flour so that in the morning the dough is easy to work. If it is too dry, the muffins end up tasting floury.
2. Mix the flour in thoroughly, and then cover the pot with a moist towel overnight.
3. In the morning, combine salt and baking soda and sprinkle over the dough. Using a large wooden spoon or your hands, turn the dough 20 to 30 times to incorporate the ingredients.
4. Place a large piece of parchment on the counter. If the dough is too sticky, sprinkle a small amount of flour over it. Divide the dough into quarters and then form each into 2 small balls. Space them evenly on the parchment, leaving them to rest and rise for approximately 30 minutes.
5. While the dough rises, preheat your oven to 325°F with the cast iron or stone pans in it.
6. After 30 minutes, remove your hot pans, lightly grease them with oil or cooking spray, and carefully transfer each ball of dough into the pans, and bake for about 8 minutes. By this time, you should be

---

PREP TIME 10–15 minutes

COOK TIME 25–30 minutes

SERVINGS Makes 8 English muffins

INGREDIENTS

½ cup sourdough starter
1 cup milk
1 tablespoon honey
2½–3 cups spelt flour
   (or 2 to 2½ cups
   whole wheat flour)
1 teaspoon salt
1 teaspoon baking soda

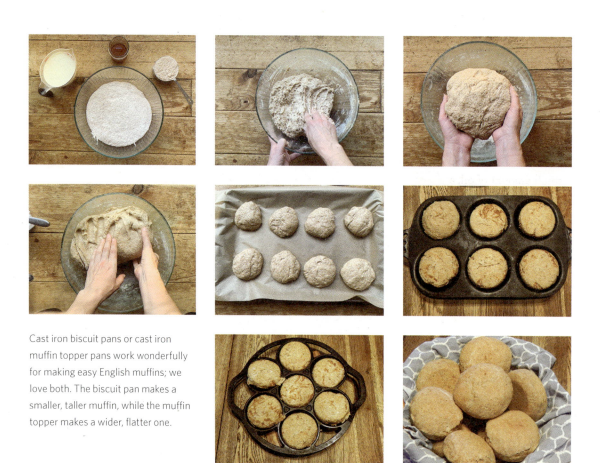

Cast iron biscuit pans or cast iron muffin topper pans work wonderfully for making easy English muffins; we love both. The biscuit pan makes a smaller, taller muffin, while the muffin topper makes a wider, flatter one.

able to gently lift the muffins and flip them in the pan. I use a knife to avoid burning my fingers.

7. Bake for 4 more minutes, then transfer the muffins to a cold baking pan or cookie sheet. This will allow their insides to finish cooking without the outsides getting too dark or burning. Put the baking pan into the oven and bake until they are sufficiently cooked, removing the pan and flipping the muffins every 5 minutes. I usually bake them 10 to 15 minutes on the pan. Once they are done, remove and place on racks to cool. Enjoy!

Oven Versus Stovetop

English muffins are traditionally made by browning each side on a skillet on the stovetop. We found we can get a similar and more consistent result with far less hands-on work using good bakeware in the oven instead.

You could do this on your stovetop if you prefer. Warm a skillet over medium heat, preferably a cast iron or similar skillet. Add a small amount of oil, and cook a few muffins until browned on one side. Flip them and cook until the other side is browned.

Sometimes the inside will need additional time to cook. If so, place the muffins on a cookie sheet and put into a preheated 325°F oven. Flip them every 5 minutes until they are fully cooked, usually 10 to 15 minutes.

MILK ALTERNATIVES

Many of our recipes use milk, but you can easily substitute similar liquids, such as buttermilk or equal parts of yogurt and water. Or, if you need a dairy-free final product, use coconut milk. Nut milks may work, but because of their fat and protein content, may require some recipe modifications.

With any substitution, remember what we said earlier about knowing your dough! Its consistency is usually more important than the measurements, so adjust flour and liquid amounts as needed.

HELL HATH NO PASTRY LIKE MY WIFE'S SCONES

PREP TIME 10–15 minutes
COOK TIME 25–30 minutes
SERVINGS Makes 12 scones

INGREDIENTS

2¼ cups spelt flour (or 1¾–2 cups whole wheat flour)
½ cup sucanat or coconut sugar
2 teaspoons cinnamon
12 tablespoons (1½ sticks) butter, lard, or leaf lard
½ cup sourdough starter
5 tablespoons (¼ cup + 1 tablespoon) milk
1 tablespoon baking powder
1 teaspoon salt

A traditional breakfast food, scones also make a nice snack or lunch dessert. They are like a sweet biscuit, sometimes with added fruit or other flavorings.

1. The night before, combine flour, sugar, and cinnamon. Using a food processor or pastry blender, cut in butter, lard, or leaf lard until pea-sized. Work the ingredients until a crumbly mixture forms.
2. Place in a medium-sized mixing bowl. Add starter and milk. Stir gently until a thick dough forms. You may need to use your hands to make sure the ingredients fully incorporate.
3. Cover the bowl with a damp cloth and set in a warm place overnight.
4. In the morning, preheat the oven to 375°F.
5. Combine baking powder and salt, and sprinkle over the dough. Gently fold the dough 10 or so times until the dry ingredients are well dispersed.
6. Divide the dough into 2 equal lumps and form the lumps into two 6-inch disks. I like to shape the disks using a 1-quart round Pyrex then removing and flattening the dough slightly with my hands. Any round bowl about the right size with a flat bottom will do.
7. Cut the disks into thirds. Cut the thirds in half, yielding 6 scones per disk.
8. Brush the scones with milk and lightly sprinkle with sucanat or another sugar.
9. Transfer the scones onto a baking sheet. You may want to use parchment to prevent the scones from sticking to the sheet. Bake for 25 to 30 minutes, rotating once after about 15 minutes.
10. The scones should be lightly brown. Allow to cool for 3 to 5 minutes, then remove from the baking sheet and enjoy.

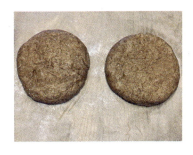
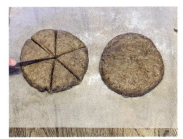
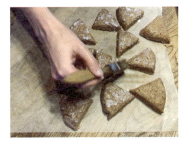
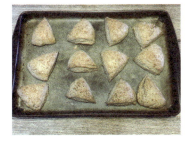
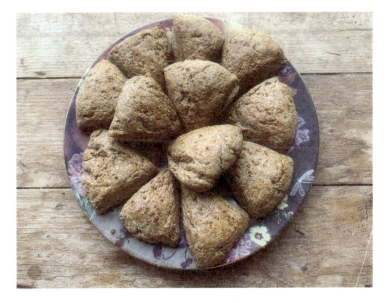

PANCAKES AND WAFFLES

What week is complete if it hasn't included pancakes?

This batter does double duty in our house — often, to speed up cooking, we will make pancakes and waffles at the same time, knocking out a few days of breakfast in a single mess-making session. Both of these freeze well.

Our pancake and waffle recipes are different than our other recipes because the starter makes up the entire base for the batter — you don't add additional flour and let it ferment! So you need a fair bit of starter, 2½ cups, for a single batch.

> **THE SAFE COOKWARE CONUNDRUM**
>
> We don't have any Teflon or similar coated cookware in our kitchen. So people often ask how we cook our waffles and pancakes. For waffles, the safest and best option on the market currently is the new ceramic-coated waffle makers. For pancakes, few things can beat a cast iron skillet or griddle. While cast iron takes time to heat up, once it is hot you can cook quickly and with better, more consistent results—well worth the short wait! Note that the cast iron griddle is also great for many other cooking needs, like hamburgers, vegetables, teriyaki chicken, and more!

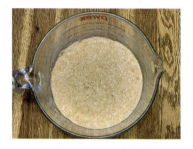
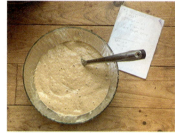
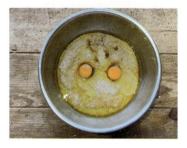
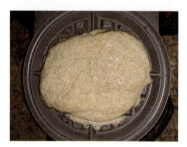

PANCAKES

You can't have breakfast and not at least occasionally have pancakes. Here is a simple recipe for when the day arises!

> **PREP TIME** 5 minutes
> **COOK TIME** 10–15 minutes
> **SERVINGS** 4
>
> **INGREDIENTS**
> 2½ cups starter
> 2 eggs
> 1½ tablespoons olive oil, melted butter, ghee, or oil/fat of your choice
> ½ tablespoon vanilla
> 1½ teaspoons baking powder
> ½ teaspoon baking soda
> 1 teaspoon salt

1. The night before, mix up enough starter (flour + water) to make 2¾ cups total starter. Allow to sit overnight.
2. In the morning, place starter in a bowl. Add eggs, olive oil (or oil of your choice), and vanilla. Mix well, making sure the eggs are fully beaten and incorporated.
3. If cooking on a cast iron skillet, start preheating it over medium heat.
4. Add baking powder, soda, and salt to mixture, stirring until incorporated.
5. Place a small amount of oil in your skillet. Using a measuring cup, scoop out about ¼ cup of batter to make medium-sized pancakes. Cook until bubbles form and pop and the top has lost some of its luster (the bottom should be lightly golden brown). Flip and cook the other side until it is golden brown (approximately 2 minutes per side).
6. Enjoy with some pastured butter and real maple syrup.
7. You can also use this recipe to make waffles, and you can use the following waffle recipe to make pancakes, just in case you were wondering!

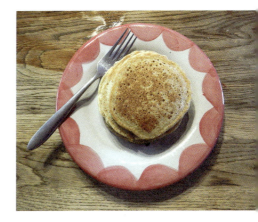

ZUCCHINI WAFFLES

PREP TIME 5–10 minutes
COOK TIME 15 minutes
SERVINGS 4 to 6

INGREDIENTS

2½ cups starter
3 eggs
¼ cup melted butter
2½ tablespoons maple syrup
½ tablespoon vanilla
¾ teaspoon cinnamon
¾ teaspoon salt
1 medium zucchini, shredded
1½ teaspoons of baking soda

Breakfast is a meal that doesn't generally include many veggies. But during zucchini and summer squash season, this is one way to turn extra zucchini (which you're likely to have on hand!) into something amazing and add some veggies into your meal plan. We'll often preserve some at the height of season by freezing shredded zucchini spread on a parchment-lined tray. Once frozen, we store it in a container or bag. Then it's on hand to add into recipes as needed.

1. The afternoon or evening before, add enough flour and water to your starter to make 2¾ cups. Go for a slightly thicker consistency.
2. In the morning, measure out 2½ cups of starter into a large bowl or pourable measuring cup. Preheat your waffle iron (or griddle if making pancakes).
3. Add eggs, melted butter, maple syrup, vanilla, cinnamon, and salt. Mix well. Fold in shredded zucchini. A food processor makes shredding much easier. Once everything is nicely mixed, add baking soda.
4. Now you are ready to make waffles or pancakes! The amount of batter and cooking time depend on your waffle iron or griddle.

> **A QUICK NOTE ON SERVING SIZE, COOKING TIME, AND WAFFLE IRONS**
>
> A few years ago, we purchased a lovely Belgian-style ceramic-coated waffle maker, which makes *massive* waffles; one is enough for two people. The ceramic coating is a safe nonstick alternative to many other options on the market, and one we highly recommend. Some people like this waffle iron so much, they own two, as its only drawback is it cooks a bit on the slow side (since the waffles are so big!). Your total cooking time will depend on how quickly your waffle iron works through the batter.

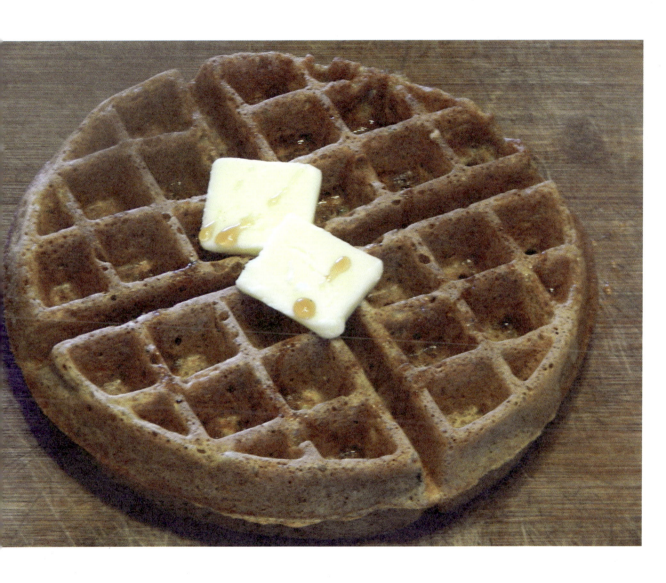

FRENCH TOAST

INGREDIENTS
1 cup milk
2 tablespoons maple syrup
A few drops vanilla
½ tablespoon Ceylon cinnamon
6 eggs
loaf of bread

Old bread — if we make a single batch, we never have this problem. But on occasion, if we make a triple, sometimes a loaf will linger on the counter or in the fridge, slowing aging and drying out, becoming unpalatable and unwanted, destined for the compost pile… unless the kids can convince their dad to turn it into French toast. This is best made with older bread since drier bread soaks up the batter better than fresh. Sometimes Jessica will make an extra loaf on purpose for a kid's requested birthday French toast breakfast or as a special treat.

1. Preheat a large cast iron skillet or griddle over medium-low heat. It takes about 5 to 10 minutes to warm ours up, giving the perfect amount of time to get the French toast ready.
2. Mix all the ingredients except the bread in a shallow Pyrex or similar baking dish. Make sure the eggs and other ingredients are thoroughly combined (we use a fork, but if you need to use a whisk or a blender, feel free).
3. Slice your bread ½ to ¾ inch thick, to your preference. We find thicker pieces hold up better. We also enjoy French toast with a soft inner layer. Soak the pieces of bread in the Pyrex for about 2 to 3 minutes the first side, then flip over and let sit for 1 more minute.
4. Turn the heat on the skillet to just above medium and add some oil (we use butter, palm shortening, or lard). Gently place a few pieces of bread into the skillet. Cook for about 2 to 3 minutes on the first side, about 2 minutes on the second. Adjust the heat as needed — thicker slices tend to do better (at least on our stove!) with slightly lower heat and longer cook time.

3

LUNCH

MAN DOES NOT live by breakfast alone, and neither does a family. Lunch rolls around roughly every 24 hours, and with it, the constant question of what will we eat? While we generally aim to make dinners large enough that leftovers can serve as the bulk of lunch, additional provisions are often needed. Also, between work, school, appointments, and everything else life throws at a family, lunch generally needs to be the easiest meal of the day. Salads and sandwiches. Crackers with freshly cut up veggies, cheese, and sausage.

BREADS

Sandwiches—there are few on-the-go-style foods as convenient. Unfortunately, there are many afflicted with poor-quality ingredients, from highly processed white bread to CAFO-raised, multisyllable-chemical-enhanced meats and cheeses, and all the sugar- and additive-laden condiments sandwiched, quite literally, in between. But sandwiches don't have to be this way. From pasture-raised meats and cheeses to a wide variety of whole grains for baking bread, you can make lunch not only delicious but also nourishing.

Bread is also the most difficult sourdough creation to produce consistently good results. Some types of breads are much easier than others. And there are some tricks to help you kick bread's butt.

IRISH SODA BREAD/ ENGLISH MUFFIN BREAD

While very similar to the English muffin recipe, the proportions are adjusted a bit to make a better bread.

1. The night before, in a large bowl, stir together starter, milk, honey, and flour. When adding flour, start with about 3½ cups. The dough will probably be very sticky and unmanageable. Add about ⅛ to ¼ cup at a time until the dough forms a nice consistency and is no longer sticky. This usually ends up being about 4 cups of spelt flour total.
2. Allow to sit for about 12 hours in a warm place.
3. In the morning, preheat oven to 350°F.
4. Work salt and soda into the dough. Fold or knead the dough lightly, until salt and baking soda are evenly distributed (about 20 to 30 folds or kneads).
5. Lightly oil your bread pan. Shape the dough into a loaf and then place into the pan. Using scissors or a sharp knife, score three deep cuts into the dough. Bake at 350°F for about 40-50 minutes.

PREP TIME 20 minutes
COOK TIME 40-50 minutes
SERVINGS Makes one large loaf

INGREDIENTS
¾ cup starter
1½ cups milk
2 tablespoons honey
3½-4½ cups spelt flour (or about 3 cups whole wheat flour)
1½ teaspoons salt
1½ teaspoons baking soda

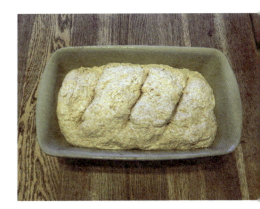

Scoring the dough helps the center of the bread to cook better and keep from cracking.

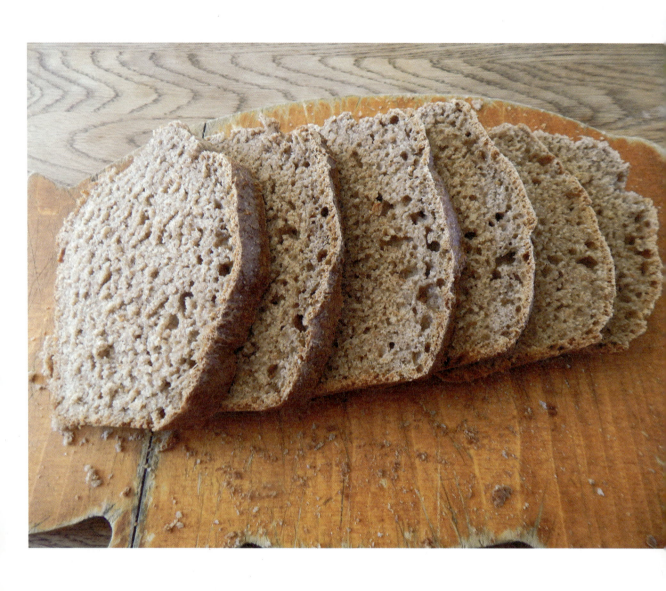

EFFICIENT KITCHEN MANAGEMENT MAKES EXCELLENT AFFORDABLE SOURDOUGH

One reason sourdough works well for us is Jessica has learned how to efficiently do the tasks. For instance, while the flour is milling twice a week for whatever is on the schedule, she not only mills the flour to feed the sourdough on the other days but also uses that time to do prep work for a recipe or cleans up in the kitchen.

This means sourdough doesn't add too much time to our already full schedule, and yet our family is able to enjoy eating it most days. As we mentioned before, Jessica typically bakes two or three days a week. We sometimes double or triple recipes so each baking session provides food for 2 to 3 days. A double recipe doesn't take much longer than a single but produces twice the food!

WHY SO MUCH BAKING SODA?

You might notice that many of our sourdough recipes use baking soda. Baking soda plays two roles in sourdough. First, it helps with rise, just like in non-sourdough recipes. Second, it is especially important when your starter is young and may still have too much twang, or strong flavor. Since baking soda is quite alkaline, it breaks down the acids that can sometimes offend eaters of sourdough, especially common in young starters and young eaters.

So don't be afraid to use baking soda to assist your success both in the kitchen and with the audience at the table!

CROUTONS
TURNING SOURDOUGH FAILURE INTO SUCCESS

PREP TIME 5 minutes
COOK TIME 12–20 minutes
SERVINGS 6 to 8

INGREDIENTS
misshapen bread (or English muffins, etc.)
½ cup (1 stick) of butter, melted
2 cloves garlic, crushed
1½ teaspoons salt

No matter what, on occasion a sourdough creation does not turn out as planned. Perhaps you were distracted or in a hurry or had a little too much help from some small hands. The temperature during the rise was too low or too much flour or liquid found its way into the dough. Such failures became the occasion for one of my favorite foods — croutons!

These croutons serve all your regular purposes: on salads and in soups, as a yummy snack, or ground up to use as breading crumbs for crusts or other dishes.

1. Preheat oven to 375°F.
2. Cut bread into ¾- to 1-inch cubes. Place them on a jelly roll or bar pan (pan with edges) or in a 9 × 13 Pyrex.
3. Mix together butter and garlic. Pour over the bread chunks. Lightly sprinkle with salt. Stir as needed to incorporate any excess butter into the bread.
4. Bake for 12 to 20 minutes, stirring every 5 minutes. Be careful not to overcook or they will become too hard to chew. Remove from oven, allow to cool, and enjoy!
5. These store excellently in a freezer. Nowadays, when we make croutons, they don't last long enough to experience its frigid depths, but once upon a smaller family, we would make two loaves at a time and have croutons on hand for a month or so during salad season.

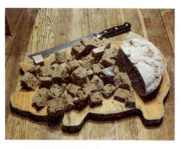

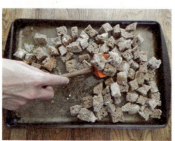

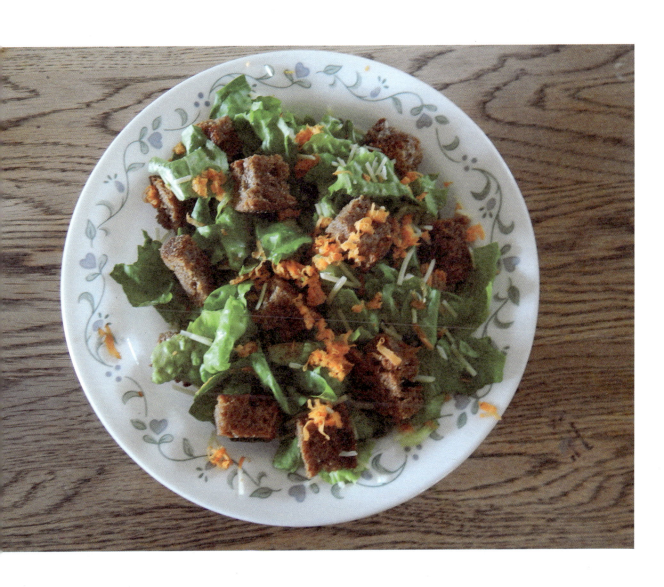

CRACKERS

Another easy lunch addition is crackers, though we often eat these as snacks or for dinner. They are amazingly expensive — basic organic crackers run about $8 per pound, while specialty ones are double that! Also, crackers are an excellent beginning recipe when your starter is young and so are you when it comes to sourdough! Since they require no rise and don't suffer from many other complications of more complex recipes, your chances of success are significantly higher.

Successful crackers require two skills: a way to easily roll them and then a method to score them so you don't end up with one big cracker.

Rolling Crackers

Two things make rolling crackers easy: a pastry roller and a pan with no edges (such as a pizza stone). We use a large Pampered Chef rectangular baking stone, but almost any edgeless pan will do. We tried recipes many years ago that had you roll the crackers and then transfer them onto the pan... the results were disastrous. I think we went five years before we were willing to try again!

Why on Earth they didn't just do the simple thing and roll out the crackers right on the baking sheet is beyond us, but at least you will know better and not need years of therapy to recover from your cracker catastrophe. If you don't have a baking sheet without edges, you can also roll them out on parchment. This requires that you carefully transfer the parchment to the baking sheet after rolling and scoring, which isn't nearly as time consuming or difficult as cutting and transferring individual crackers.

Scoring Crackers

One of the main difficulties with crackers is how to get them to crack apart evenly. It is a good deal easier than you realize once you know the secret. First, you should score the rolled out dough right before

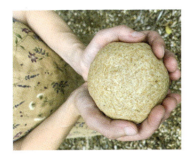
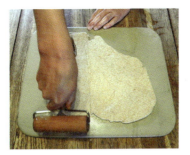
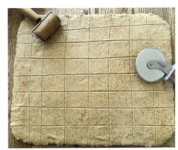
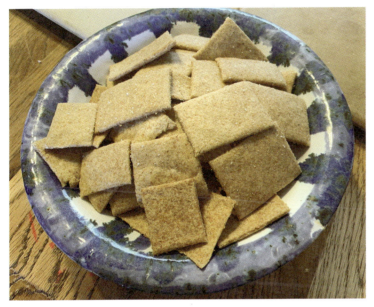

the crackers go into the oven. Second, you can use a pizza cutter to make this much easier. If you don't have one, any knife does fine; it is just harder to get straight, long cuts. A cutter also lets you customize cracker size, or even get a little artistic — our kids always get a kick out of when Jessica uses a ravioli or similar cutter to create decorative patterns along the edges.

By scoring the crackers before cooking, they naturally break apart or become very weak along the lines as they bake. Once cooled, they easily separate.

BASIC CRACKERS

> **PREP TIME** 20 minutes
> **COOK TIME** 20 minutes
> **SERVINGS** 6 to 8; Yields two large trays of thin crackers or two medium-sized trays of thicker crackers.
>
> **INGREDIENTS**
> 1 cup sourdough starter
> ¼ cup palm shortening or lard
> ½ teaspoon salt
> 1¼ cup spelt flour (or 1 cup whole wheat flour), divided

Now for the recipe! This is adapted from one we first saw many years ago on The Kitchen Stewardship website.

1. In a bowl, mix thoroughly starter and palm shortening or lard to make a somewhat watery dough. Combine ¼ cup whole wheat or spelt flour and ½ teaspoon salt and mix into the dough.

2. Add enough flour to make the dough stiff — for whole wheat, it takes about ¾ cup; for spelt, a hair less than 1 cup. Since you will be rolling the dough out thinly, it is very important that it is firm enough to work. Allow to sit at room temperature for 7 to 12 hours.

3. Preheat your oven to 350°F. Take about half of the dough and roll it out on your baking pan or parchment, to a thin, uniform thickness, depending on your preference. It is very important that the entire tray be about the same thickness, or some will burn and others may end up undercooked. Add more dough as necessary to fill the baking sheet. This recipe usually fills one large baking sheet with some left over. We roll this out onto a second baking sheet, taking care to keep the thickness uniform, especially on the edges. If the crackers along the edges are too thin, they will quickly burn.

4. Once rolled, the crackers are ready for scoring. Again, the size is up to you. Uniformity does not matter when scoring, so feel free to be creative and do as you please! Sprinkle the crackers with salt if desired.

5. Bake for 15 to 20 minutes, until the crackers are lightly browned. Note that very thin crackers can go from almost done to burnt very quickly! Remove from the oven. You can cool them on the pan, but keep in mind that they may continue cooking if the pan holds heat well (like stoneware does); watch to make sure they don't get too done. If you are using stoneware or similar cookware, the crackers will crisp up a bit more during this time. You can also remove them immediately from the pan to cool.

6. Transfer to a bowl or dish and enjoy.

Beyond Basic Crackers

Note that the crackers don't have much flavor of their own, especially if using standard wheat flour. Spelt, kamut, and einkorn all give far more flavor. Also, this recipe is a great base for all sorts of additions—tomato, basil, rosemary, grated cheese — the sky is the limit for where you go from here!

> **FREEZING DOUGH**
>
> A friend of ours used to sell frozen sourdough cracker dough, which many people loved to purchase from her. You can freeze the dough for this recipe, and for a number of others. This can let you make a double or triple batch, and then save some dough for later when you are ready to bake more, instead of starting from scratch, like when you get surprise visitors or just need a meal option that is slightly faster to prepare.
>
> All you need to do is, in the last steps, instead of adding the final ingredients like baking soda and salt, you take the dough, place it in an appropriate container, and pop it into the freezer. Before using, it is best to thaw the dough in the fridge, rather than at room temperature.

ARTISAN SPELT BREAD

Few foods have as many books, websites, recipes, and as much fanfare as artisan breads. Many recipes are quite particular, requiring very precise conditions and measurements to achieve the desired results. If you have the interest, it is a fun and challenging area to explore. We wanted to include a simpler approach to a whole grain artisan bread for you to try and enjoy.

Most artisan breads use at least some white flour. With this recipe, we have been able to get a good rise, a fairly open crumb, as well as great texture and flavor, while sticking to only whole grain flour.

For this recipe, you want your starter as active as possible. To ensure this, I like to feed it frequently for 2 to 3 days before making this particular bread. Although we usually use spelt to feed our starter, I have found that whole wheat flour gives a better result. Actually, we go even further and make a "super starter" for this recipe which we'll tell you all about in the sidebar below.

Because this dough is quite moist, it helps immensely to wet your hands before handling it. If you are not familiar with the terms and techniques in this recipe, you can find demonstration videos on the internet. One I especially like is made by Homemade Food Junkie, called "Beginner Artisan Sourdough Bread Recipe," which is available on Youtube.

For optimal results, supercharge your starter for 2 or more feedings before mixing the dough for this recipe by discarding all but 50 grams (3 tablespoons) of starter and adding 50 grams (7 to 8 tablespoons) of sifted, debranned wheat flour (see sidebar) and 50 grams (3½ tablespoons) of water. On the morning before, again discard all but 50 grams of starter and add 50 grams sifted whole wheat flour and 50 grams of water. When making the super starter for this recipe we like to measure by weight, but if you don't have a good food scale, feed your starter to make a slightly thicker than normal starter.

CREATING SUPER STARTER

Starter made with whole grains is strong, but may you need to supercharge your starter, especially for more difficult tasks like bread. The easiest way to do this if you mill your own grains is to use a small strainer to remove the bigger bits of bran — the hard outer layer of cereal grains — from the germ. We don't use our flour sifter because its holes are big enough to let the bran fall right through. Straining the larger flecks of bran will leave behind a much lighter and whiter flour that will have a lot more rising power than its 100% whole grain counterpart. I like to do this by pushing the freshly milled flour through a fine strainer using a spoon. Stir a small amount of flour in the strainer vigorously but being careful to keep the bran in the strainer. The lighter flour will fall through. This works great to make a potent starter with extra rising power. Don't be tempted to supercharge your whole grain starter using store-bought all purpose flour though! It is too different from the whole grain flour you usually feed it with, and it will take a while to adjust and produce good sourdough activity and rise. On the other hand, if you already have a healthy bubbly starter made from all purpose flour, feel free to use that with our recipes. It should work fine, and this particular recipe only calls for ¼ cup of starter, so the resulting loaf would be over 95% whole grain.

You might wonder why most bread is made with de-branned/all purpose flour. The bran contains fatty acids, along with a number of other nutrients, that go rancid fairly quickly once milled. So one reason among many was to keep bread tasting better longer. This is also partly why so many modern foods like bread are fortified; that is, vitamins and minerals (often synthetic) are added to replace what was taken out earlier. Doesn't make any sense to me, at least. Why not just, whenever possible, leave all the good stuff nature already packaged together together?

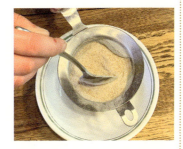

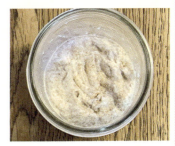

Once the dough is ready, you will stretch and fold the dough several times. As you do so, the dough's texture will change, creating a stretchier easier-to-handle dough.

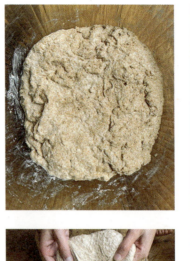
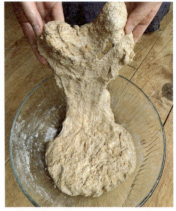
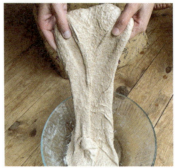
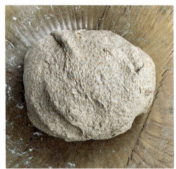

INGREDIENTS

5½ cups spelt flour

2 cups filtered water

¼ cup super starter

½ tablespoon salt

Now, for the recipe. Our artisan bread is made out of just flour, water, and salt, and you'll be amazed with the results. The procedure has more steps than most of our recipes, but if you follow them, we're confident even a beginner will make great whole grain artisan bread.

Since you want to make sure you use the starter at its peak, plan to keep an eye on it and to make the dough about 6 to 8 hours after feeding it. When the starter is ready, it should be domed on top, about double in size, with lots of bubbles and air pockets all around. Make sure you use it before it flattens on top, which is a sign you missed its most active window. If you did miss this, feed it again and wait until it is at its most active stage again. We find that beginning Step 1 in the mid to late afternoon works best so the dough is ready to go in the fridge overnight.

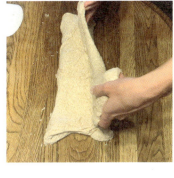 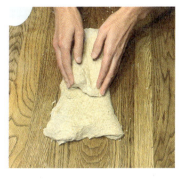 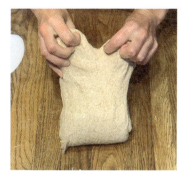
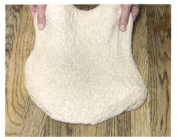 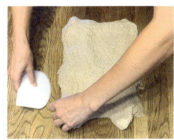 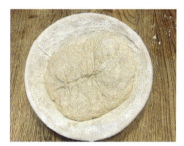

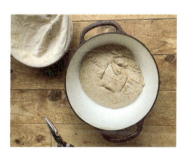

Wet hands will allow you to carefully and effectively shape the dough for the final loaf.

1. Combine ingredients in a large mixing bowl to form a wet dough. Let it rest in the mixing bowl for 30 minutes.
2. Then use two hands to grab the dough on the right side, stretch it as far as possible, and fold it over to the left side. Rotate the bowl 90 degrees and stretch and fold from that side. Keep rotating the bowl, stretching and folding until you have done it from four sides. Cover the bowl with a damp cloth and let it sit for 30 minutes.
3. Repeat the stretch and fold on all four sides like you did before. Cover and let it sit another 30 minutes.
4. Repeat the stretch and fold two more times for a total of 4 sets separated by 30 minutes. Place the dough in a covered bowl to rest and rise for 1 hour. Then place the entire mixing bowl into a plastic grocery bag. Tie the bag shut and refrigerate overnight.
5. In the morning, take the bowl from the fridge and let it sit for about 2 hours until it reaches room temperature. Remove the bag and place the dough on a clean unfloured surface, such as a counter or table.

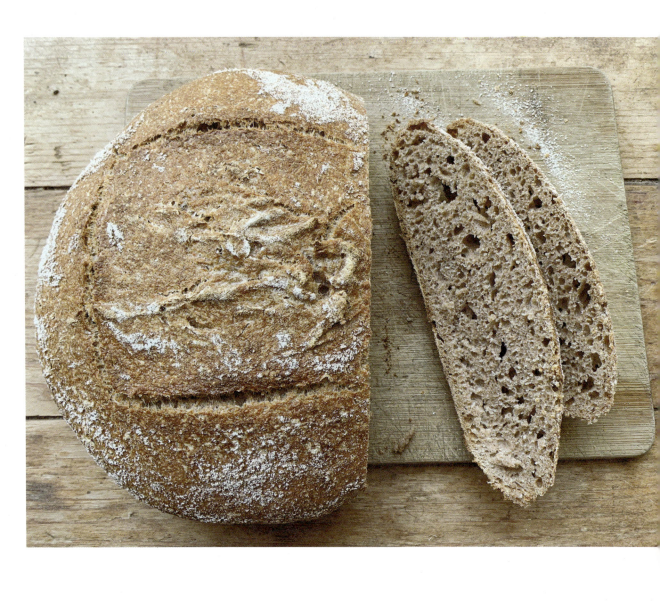

Do not use parchment, or it will stick. Use a dough scraper to gently form it into a ball/mound by scraping around the dough at its base.

6. Sprinkle the top with flour and let it sit for 20 minutes. Position the dough scraper under the dough and flip it onto the floured side.

7. To shape the loaf, wet your hands and pull the dough into a rectangular shape from the edges. Take the right side of the dough and pull it over toward the left about ⅓ of the way. Then take the left side and pull it toward the right side all the way over to the fold (which is now the edge of the loaf on the right side).

8. Now you have a long folded dough. Take one of the short ends and fold it into the middle. Finally, take the other short end and fold it over and wrap the dough around on all sides and form a seam on the underside of the ball. If you haven't shaped a loaf this way before, the video I mentioned above is very helpful.

9. Line a strainer, medium-sized bowl, or banneton (also known as a proofing basket) with a cloth and sprinkle with flour. White rice flour works the best to ensure your dough doesn't stick, but you can also use whatever flour you have on hand. You can wet the cloth and really work the flour into the cloth as well to help. Make sure you use enough flour so that the dough won't stick when you remove it for baking.

10. Cover and refrigerate for 2 hours. After 1 hour and 15 minutes, put an empty Dutch oven in the oven and preheat at 450°F for 45 minutes.

11. Once the dough is ready and the oven and Dutch oven are preheated, remove the Dutch oven. Remove the banneton from the fridge and carefully transfer the loaf into the Dutch oven. A dough scraper can help if it sticks at all. Working quickly, score the top of your loaf with a razor blade, put the lid on the Dutch oven, and bake for 30 minutes. Take the lid off and continue baking 10 to 15 more minutes until the loaf is nicely browned on top.

12. Remove the bread from the pan and allow to cool on a rack for 2 hours.

> **WET HANDS MAKE WORKING DOUGH GO WELL**
> A quick tip: When you need to work dough by hand, first rinse your hands with filtered water and leave them damp. This keeps it from sticking to your hands and makes working it worlds easier.

DINNER

INTERESTINGLY, DINNER IS the meal when we generally eat the least sourdough. Between squash, potatoes, sweet potatoes, rice, and so many other starchy vegetable options, sourdough faces stiff dinnertime competition. But there are certain meals that just aren't the same without particular traditional pairings: biscuits with rice and gravy, rolls with roast beef, chicken pot pie with a deep, rich, buttery crust. Sourdough definitely has a place, even at a crowded dinner table!

BISCUITS

What dinner, regular or holiday, doesn't benefit from a biscuit? Paired with stews or soups, or as a side with jam or jelly, a biscuit is a basic easy-to-make enjoyment to add to your repertoire. Our recipe is adapted from one we found on the Cultures for Health website.

PREP TIME 15 minutes
COOK TIME 20-30 minutes
SERVINGS 12 to 14, depending on size

INGREDIENTS
½ cup (1 stick) butter
2½ cups spelt or whole wheat flour
½ cup sourdough starter
1 tablespoon honey
1 cup buttermilk or milk
¾ teaspoon salt
1 teaspoon baking powder
1 teaspoon baking soda

1. On the night before, cut butter into flour with a food processor or pastry cutter. Stir in starter, honey, and milk.
2. Add more flour (usually around 1 to 4 tablespoons) to make a good dough. Keep in mind that you will need to roll it out before cutting the biscuits, so aim for a dough that has just enough flour to roll out without being a sticky mess. You can add slightly more later if necessary, so it is best to err on the side of too little than too much.
3. Cover and allow to sit for 7 to 12 hours.
4. In the morning, preheat oven to 400°F.
5. Combine salt, baking powder, and baking soda in a small bowl. Sprinkle the mixture a little at a time over the dough, then fold the dough. Repeat until the mixture is incorporated, about 20 folds.
6. Roll dough out to approximately ½ inch thick. Cut into 2- to 3-inch rounds — the top of a pint or similar size jar works well for this task. Reform the excess, roll out to ½ inch thick, and cut additional biscuits. Form any excess dough by hand into the last biscuit.
7. Place the biscuits on a cookie sheet or biscuit pan and bake for 20 to 30 minutes, until the tops are golden brown.

CUT SQUARE BISCUITS AND SAVE TIME

Another option for biscuits is to square cut the dough, a technique we learned from our friend Dann Reid. Roll out the dough into a rectangle, straighten all the edges to ensure an even rise, and then cut in half across the middle. Make all cuts straight down; do not saw. Cut each half into your desired quantity and size of biscuits. With this technique there is no waste or excess dough to reroll like you have when cutting rounds.

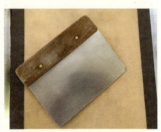

DANN REID.

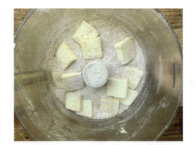
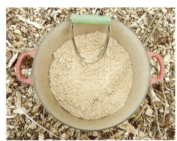
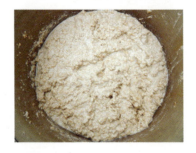
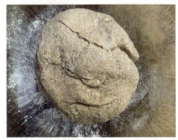
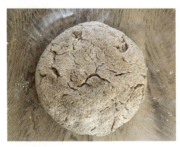
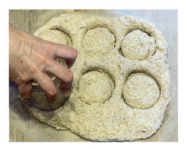
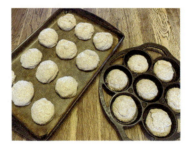

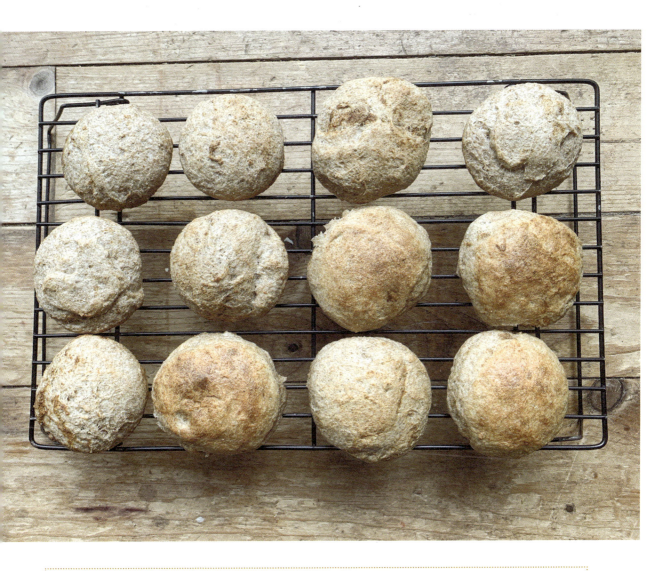

WHAT'S THE DIFFERENCE BETWEEN A BISCUIT, ROLL, MUFFIN, AND SO MANY OTHER BAKED GOODS?

Have you ever wondered why there are so many baked goods and what makes each different? It is all about which ingredients are or are not included and how the dough is formed. Rolls are literally rolled, while biscuits are generally cut from the dough or spooned. Rolls use yeast, while biscuits use baking powder. English muffins contain milk but little to no fat, but some other creations contain fat but no milk. It is the unique interplay of different ingredients and incorporation methods that gives each baked good its unique texture, taste, and place at our table!

ROLLS

PREP TIME 20 minutes (10 night before, 10 morning of)

COOK TIME 20–30 minutes

SERVINGS Makes 12 large or 18 medium rolls

INGREDIENTS

¾ cup starter
1½ cups milk
2½ tablespoons honey
2½ tablespoons melted butter
4 to 5 cups spelt flour
1½ teaspoons salt
1½ teaspoons baking soda

There are few foods as quintessential and essential as dinner rolls. So many meals seem incomplete without them, and what holiday occasion and properly provisioned table lacks them? Sopping up the leftovers of soups and stews, or serving as a scrumptious sponge to clean up drippings off your plate. Dinner would be emptier and dishes harder without these adorning your table!

This recipe makes delicious dinner rolls or, if you make them larger, excellent hotdog and hamburger buns.

1. On the night before, mix starter, milk, honey, butter, and flour together, starting with 4 cups of flour. Keep adding flour, one tablespoon at a time, until you have a slightly sticky dough. Place dough into a bowl, cover with a damp cloth, and allow to sit for 8 to 12 hours.
2. In the morning, preheat your oven to 350°F.
3. Combine salt and soda, and sprinkle over dough. Work into the dough by carefully folding it 20 or so times. It is best to break up any clumps of baking soda before you sprinkle it onto the surface.
4. With wet hands, separate the dough in half. Separate these into thirds. For large rolls like hamburger buns, separate in half again. For dinner rolls, separate into three equal portions again.
5. Place rolls in a greased glass pan (two 8 × 8 pans or a 9 × 13 pan should fit all the rolls). Allow to sit for 30 minutes to rise.
6. Bake for 20 to 30 minutes, until they are browned on the top and sides. Remove from oven, cool in the pans for about 5 minutes, then place on a cooling rack or enjoy warm.

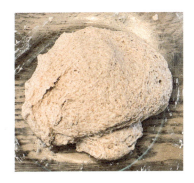 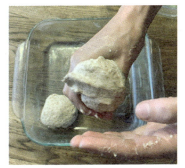 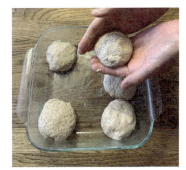
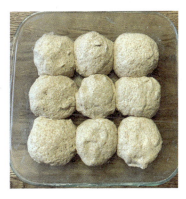 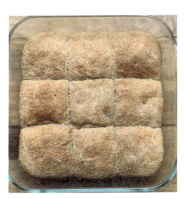

EMPANADAS

PREP TIME 1.5 hours
COOK TIME 1 hour
SERVINGS Makes about 24 empanadas

INGREDIENTS

2 pounds ground beef
1 teaspoon ground cumin or cumin seeds, divided
1 onion, chopped
2 bunches green onions or 2 tablespoons chives, chopped
2 red or green peppers, seeded and chopped
4 to 5 cloves garlic, peeled and smashed or finely chopped
3 carrots, peeled and grated
2 tablespoons parsley (fresh or dried)
¼ cup cilantro, chopped
1 cup cooked peas
1½ cups cooked brown or white rice (½ cup dry rice)
Sea salt and pepper
2–3 tablespoons olive oil

This is quite possibly my favorite easy out-of-the-fridge-or-freezer food. While in the dinner section, these are an absolutely amazing on-the-go lunch option. Two or three empanadas make a decent meal all by themselves, no sides needed. These freeze excellently as well, so you can do a large batch and have them for that emergency lunch or dinner option that lets you skip having to eat fast food. Also note this recipe scales easily; we normally double it.

Our original empanadas were made using Sally Fallon's recipe from *The Nourishing Traditions* cookbook. Our current recipe is still very similar, with some tweaks and adaptations, especially to the dough that forms the crust into which all the empanada goodness goes. The original is a fermented yogurt dough, whereas this is a true sourdough crust.

One note, this is the most time-consuming recipe in the entire book. Using a food processor or similar appliance to chop and grate ingredients, especially if you are doing a large batch, is very helpful. You can soak and then cook the rice and peas the day before.

We usually do this recipe over two days: the first day, we make the filling and crust; the second day, we do the rolling, filling, and baking. The great thing is that, once the work is done, you will have lots of empanadas on hand to eat over a few days or freeze.

1. In a skillet over medium heat, sauté ground beef, stirring often until cooked through and lightly browned. If the ground beef is low in fat, add oil to prevent burning. Season with ½ teaspoon cumin, sea salt, and pepper to taste.

2. In a separate skillet, sauté onions and peppers in olive oil until soft (approximately 15 minutes). While they cook, peel and grate the carrots (we use a food processor for quick grating), press the garlic, cook the rice and peas, and chop the remaining vegetables (parsley and cilantro).

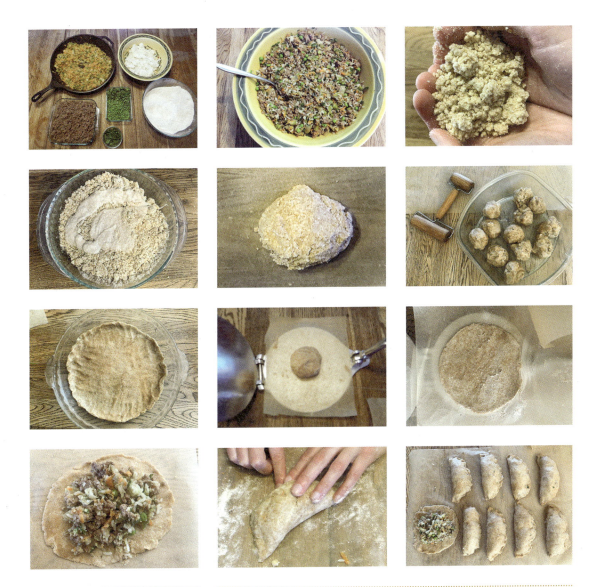

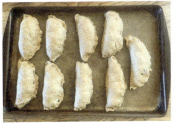

BE FLEXIBLE WITH YOUR FILLINGS

For empanadas, the vegetables in the filling are more like suggestions than rules. I (John) don't tolerate corn well, which is why this rather common ingredient to this dish is missing. Feel free to adjust the vegetable mix according to your preferences and the possibilities your particular location and season presents.

PREP TIME 15 minutes
COOK TIME 20–40 minutes
SERVINGS Makes 2 pie crusts or 12 empanadas. Double this recipe if you want to make 24 empanadas.

INGREDIENTS
2 cups spelt flour
½ teaspoon salt
1 cup (2 sticks) cold unsalted butter
¾ cup sourdough starter

TORTILLA PRESS TIPS
When using the press, we cut two small pieces of parchment paper just larger than the press's surface. Place one sheet on the bottom, plop a piece of dough in the center, then place the second sheet on top. With your hand, gently press down the dough ball, then finish with the tortilla press. You should quickly and easily form nice, relatively round crusts.

3. Add the carrots and garlic to the onions and peppers, along with another ½ teaspoon cumin and salt and pepper to taste. Sauté for another 5 minutes. Remove from heat. Allow to cool.
4. In a large bowl, thoroughly mix everything — all the vegetables, the ground beef, and rice. Don't forget the parsley and cilantro. Place in a container and refrigerate overnight. Now it is time to prepare the crust.

EMPANADA CRUST

1. The night before baking the empanadas, combine flour, salt, and butter in a food processor. Process until pea-sized crumbs form, usually 30 to 40 seconds. If you don't have a food processor, slice cold butter and then cut into flour using a pastry blender.
2. Add starter, mix lightly, and then pour onto parchment. Gather and knead to form into a dough. If it doesn't incorporate into a dough, continue to add starter, 1 tablespoon at a time, until the dough forms. Place in a bowl, cover with a damp cloth, and leave in a warm spot overnight.
3. Preheat the oven to 350°F. Take the dough and divide it into 12 equal-sized balls. Lightly flour some parchment or your work surface.
4. Take a single ball and flatten it slightly by hand first. Then use a pastry roller to roll out the dough into a medium-thickness crust. It will take a few tries to get used to making these. You can also press them with a tortilla press — it will make this part much easier and faster.
5. Once your dough is rolled to an appropriate thickness, scoop a scant ½ cup of the filling and place it in the middle. Carefully enclose the filling by folding the dough in half and pinching the sides together. As you finish preparing the empanadas, place them on a cookie sheet. Bake in batches until lightly browned, about 20 minutes. If you happen to have extra filling, freeze it for later use. It is also delicious on a salad or tortilla.
6. Enjoy these fresh out of the oven or allow to cool and freeze to have on hand for a delicious ready-made meal on a busy day.

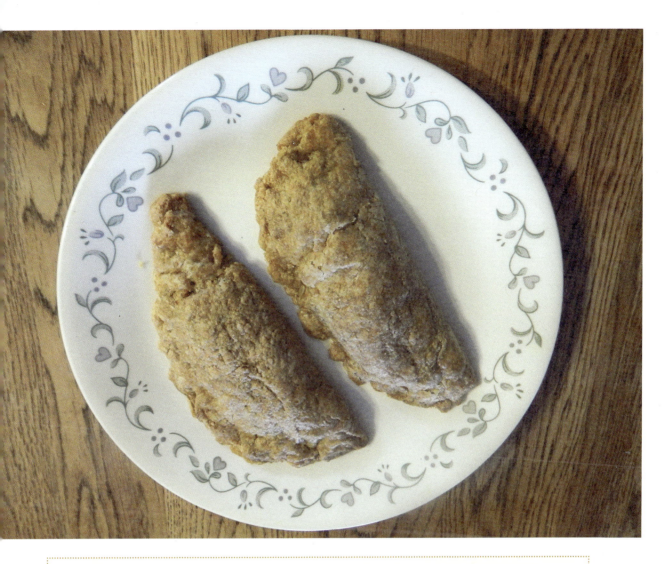

PIE CRUSTS

The pie crust recipe we have provided is made without sugar. It can also be used for chicken pot pie as well as sweet pies and pastries. If you are making a dessert, you will likely want a sweeter crust. Just add a tablespoon of sugar to the above recipe and enjoy!

As a kid, one of my favorite treats was a dish my grandma called cinnamon pie crust. She would take any extra dough left over from making pies, roll it out thinly, sprinkle it with cinnamon and sugar, and then bake it until crisp. If you end up with extra dough, you can freeze it or make this simple snack.

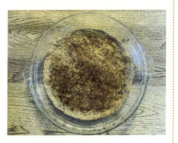

SNACKS AND SPECIAL TREATS

MUFFINS

"Is there anything I can eat?" We probably hear this petition thirty to three hundred times a day — at home, in the car, after judo, 15 minutes after lunch, 20 minutes before dinner. Kids get hungry far more often than I remember as a child. While our kids eat a fair amount of fruit and vegetables, we need to have some other options to slow them down. And what book about baking is complete without a muffin recipe, especially a blueberry muffin one?

BASIC MUFFINS

1. On the night before, mix starter, butter, and honey well. Add flour and mix in water. Cover with a damp cloth. Allow to sit in a warm place overnight.
2. In the morning, preheat your oven to 350°F. While it is preheating, add eggs, salt, baking soda, and cinnamon to your batter, stirring well until they are thoroughly incorporated. This may take a little elbow grease, but try not to overwork the batter. Jessica will often use her hands to ensure the batter mixes well.
3. Bake for 12 to 15 minutes, until the muffins are golden brown and no longer glossy on top. You can also stick a long toothpick into the muffins; it should come out clean if they are fully cooked.
4. Removed from the oven and allow the muffins to sit for 5 or so minutes, then transfer to a wire rack to cool.

> **PREP TIME** 15 minutes
> **COOK TIME** 15–20 minutes
> **SERVINGS** Makes approximately 12 muffins
>
> **INGREDIENTS**
> ¾ cup starter
> ⅓ cup melted butter
> ⅓ cup honey
> 1½ cups spelt flour (or 1¼ cup whole wheat flour)
> ¼ cup water
> 2 eggs
> 1 teaspoon salt
> 1¼ teaspoons baking soda
> 2 teaspoons cinnamon (optional)

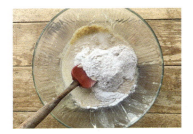
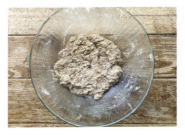
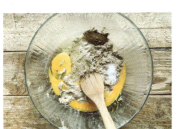
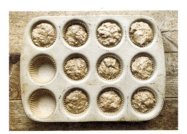
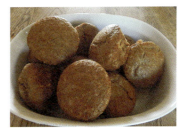

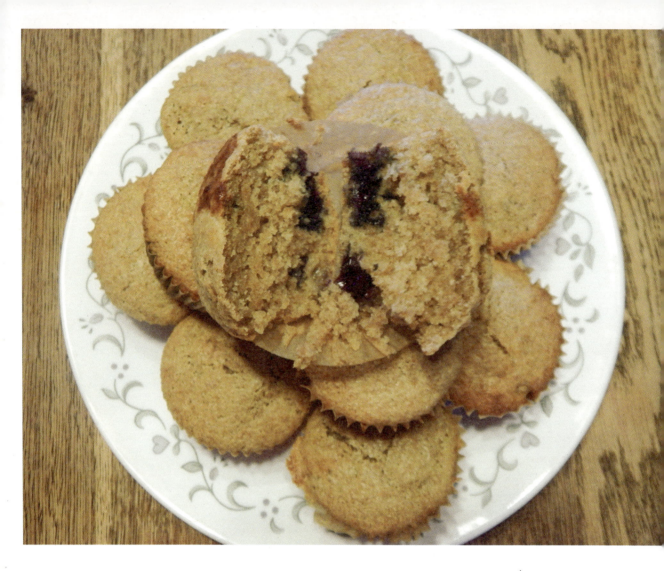

Blueberry Muffins

Basic muffins are marvelous, but I (John) think they marry well with various fruits, especially fresh or frozen local blueberries.

To make the basic muffins blue, omit the cinnamon and add 1 cup of blueberries to the batter with the other morning ingredients. If using frozen berries, increase your oven temperature to 375°F.

HOW TO CONVERT STANDARD RECIPES TO SOURDOUGH

Do you have a family favorite recipe that you would like to make work with your sourdough? It often isn't too hard. A number of our recipes were originally regular or Sue Gregg-style (blender batter) dishes that we adapted to sourdough.

There are a few basic tips that will help you make the transition. First, you want to keep close to the same amount of flour and liquid in the recipe. For our starter, 1 tablespoon of water plus 1½ tablespoons of flour yields just over 1¼ tablespoons of starter. For the mathematically astute, you probably noticed that you end up with slightly *less* total volume when you combine the flour with water. This means that if we are using 1 cup of starter, it is slightly less than 1 cup of liquid and slightly more than 1 cup of flour to subtract from the recipe.

This lets you calculate new ingredient proportions, which we can then work from based on your results. Note, it will still take a few attempts to determine your final amounts — this just helps you find a good starting point.

For example, our original muffin recipe called for 1 cup of buttermilk and 2¼ cups of flour. Since we use ¾ cup of starter, we subtracted from the recipe ⅔ cup of liquid (slightly less than ¾ cup) and ⅞ cup of flour (slightly more than ¾ cup). So, we want to add ⅓ cup liquid and 1⅜ cup of flour to the starter for the converted recipe.

ORIGINAL LESS	STARTER (¾ CUP TOTAL)	NEW STARTING PROPORTIONS
1 cup liquid	⅔ cup liquid	⅓ cup liquid
2¼ cups flour	⅞ cup flour	1⅜ cups flour

Note that oils or sweeteners are generally not considered liquids in a recipe. Those will stay the same in your new version.

The above became the starting point for the sourdough version. But after a few tries, we lowered the amount of liquid to ¼ cup and increased the flour to 1½ cups. Keep in mind the consistency of the batter or dough from the original recipe and work with your adjustments to match it. As the sourdough starter ferments, it tends to become a bit thinner, and sometimes this means your sourdough adaptation may need slightly less total liquid and a tad more flour than the original recipe. Keep experimenting until you get it right. Your first try may not be a winner, but it has generally yielded an acceptable to more than acceptable first attempt that no one complains about eating.

CAST IRON SKILLET CINNAMON ROLLS

PREP TIME 30 minutes
COOK TIME 25–35 minutes
SERVINGS Makes 9 to 12 rolls

INGREDIENTS
½ cup (1 stick) butter
3 cups spelt flour (or 2½ cups whole wheat flour)
½ cup sourdough starter
1 tablespoon honey
1 cup milk
¾ teaspoon salt
¾ teaspoon baking soda
1 teaspoon baking powder

If muffins are an easy mainstay, cinnamon rolls are a celebration kind of treat. Not an everyday item, but something to break out around holidays and other special occasions, or just as a special treat whenever wanted! We adapted this recipe from one at Cultures for Health — when we saw that their recipe was cooked in a cast iron skillet we figured it would be a good one. This version uses only whole grains and sugars.

1. On the night before, slice butter into ½ tablespoon size pieces. Cut it into 2½ cups of spelt or whole wheat flour. Our favorite way to do this is with a food processor, but you can also do it in a bowl, using a pastry knife.
2. In a large bowl, combine sourdough starter, honey, and milk, stirring well. Now, add the flour and butter mixture and stir. The final consistency should be wet and sticky.
3. If you are using spelt flour, add ½ cup to make a soft dough. If you are using whole wheat flour, you will not need to add any flour unless the dough is extremely sticky. Whichever flour you are using, keep in mind that, in the morning, you will have to knead and shape the dough. If it is too sticky, you won't be able to work with it, but if it is too dry or floury, the end result won't rise correctly or taste as fantastic.
4. Put the dough in a bowl and cover with a damp cloth. Allow it to sit overnight a warm place (about 12 hours).
5. In the morning, combine salt, baking soda, and baking powder and sprinkle over the dough. Knead 20 to 30 times, until these are well incorporated.
6. It is now time to shape the dough. I prefer to do this on parchment laid on a counter or table. You can also use a Silpat or just a clean counter or tabletop. Because the dough is soft, it tends to stick to the rolling pin, so instead, I use my hands to gently press it into a rectangle, about ½ inch thick. Let the dough rest while you make the filling.

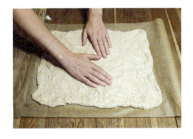
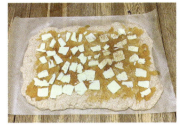

Our honey filling is made with honey, butter, and cinnamon. It makes the pastry extra gooey and is our favorite.

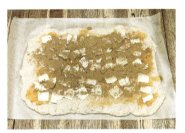
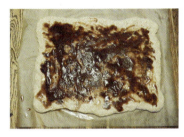

Our whole sugar filling uses coconut sugar (or sucanat), butter, and cinnamon and is also delicious and less messy to work with.

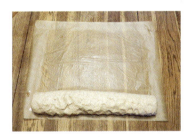
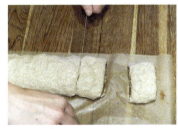

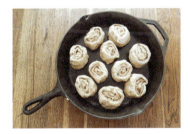
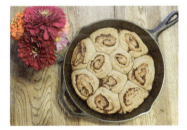

Snacks and Special Treats

7. Prepare and add filling to dough. At this point, you can add ingredients, such as raisins, chopped walnuts or pecans, or whatever else floats your cinnamon roll filling fancy. I (John) have a soft spot for walnuts or pecans.
8. Now, starting at the top, carefully roll the dough longways into a log.
9. How do you make the individual rolls? Here's a trick courtesy of Sue Gregg. Take a clean piece of unflavored dental floss, about 14 to 18 inches. Lift up one end of the roll, and slide the floss underneath, about 1½ inches from the end. Cross the floss over itself and then pull, cleanly cutting your first roll. It sounds tricky, but is quite easy once you do it a few times. Repeat until the entire log is cut into individual rolls, about 9 to 12.
10. Place the individual rolls, cut side up, into a greased 10- or 12-inch cast iron skillet. You can also use a greased 9 × 13 Pyrex. Allow to rise for approximately 30 minutes. During this time, preheat the oven to 350°F.
11. Bake the rolls until the tops are golden brown, about 25 to 35 minutes.

FILLING OPTIONS

While, traditionally, cinnamon rolls are made with sugar, and more recently, with honey, there are many sweetener options for you to use based on your particular preferences.

Whole Sugar Filling

Ingredients

½ cup (1 stick) butter

2 teaspoons cinnamon

½ cup plus 2 tablespoons coconut sugar, sucanat, or brown sugar.

To make the whole sugar filling, start by gently melting the butter. Add cinnamon and coconut sugar, sucanat, or brown sugar and combine.

Put filling directly onto the center of the dough rectangle. Spread outward in all directions, leaving about ¾ to 1 inch uncovered on all sides

Christmas Morning Filling

Ingredients

¼ cup sucanat

⅜ cup date syrup

2 teaspoons cinnamon

½ cup (1 stick) butter, sliced

After we finished our first draft, we played around a bit more with a number of recipes. On Christmas morning we made the cinnamon rolls with a new filling. So here is that option, as I (John) enjoyed it immensely.

To make the Christmas morning filling, sprinkle the sucanat on the dough and drizzle the date syrup over that. Place the sliced butter on the sweeteners and sprinkle cinnamon on top.

Honey Filling

Ingredients

¾ cup honey

½ cup (1 stick) butter, sliced thin

1 tablespoon cinnamon

To make the honey filling, simply spread the honey across the pressed dough, leaving about 1 inch or so on all sides. Place the sliced butter across the honey. Sprinkle cinnamon on top.

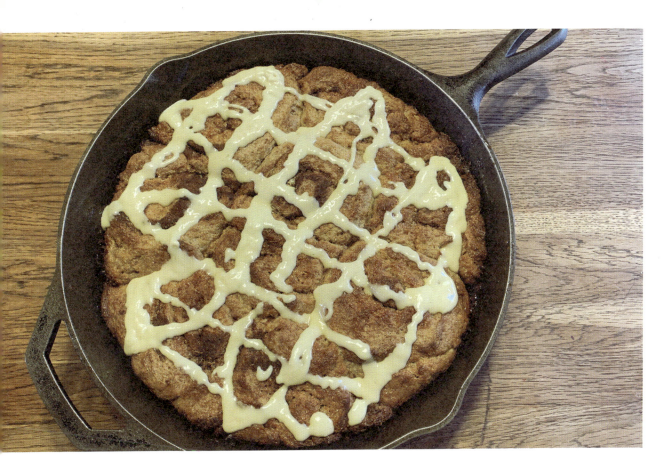

CREAM CHEESE FROSTING

The above recipe may strike some as a tad undersweet without frosting. Since cinnamon rolls are usually frosted, while we don't generally eat them with it, we felt including this frosting option was important. Usually, frosting is loaded with powdered sugar, but if you want a healthier option, try this wonderful recipe from The Adventure Bite website. It is easy to make and delicious.

INGREDIENTS

2 8-ounce packages
   cream cheese
½ cup (1 stick) salted butter
½ cup maple syrup
1 tablespoon vanilla extract

1. Bring cream cheese and butter to room temperature. Beat together until smooth. Add syrup and vanilla extract while mixing slowly. Spread or pipe frosting over the cinnamon rolls. Refrigerate until ready to use.

CINNAMON RAISIN BREAD

PREP TIME 30 minutes
BAKE TIME 30-40 minutes
SERVINGS Makes 1 medium sized loaf

INGREDIENTS
⅔ cup sourdough starter
⅔ cup milk
2 tablespoons honey
2 tablespoons melted butter
1½ teaspoons cinnamon
2½ to 3½ cups flour (usually around 3 cups)
3 tablespoons coconut sugar, sucanat, or brown sugar
1 tablespoon cinnamon
1 teaspoon salt
1 teaspoon baking soda
¾ cup raisins

I (John) generally don't like cooked fruit, but this recipe is the delicious exception to the rule. This bread is wonderful fresh, toasted, or turned into French toast. We love it at breakfast, lunch, dinner… or as I type this, I am going to get myself another piece as a snack, since writing about it made me hungry for more!

It takes a bit more time to make, but the end result is worth it.

1. The night before, mix starter, milk, honey, butter, and 1½ tablespoon of cinnamon together in a glass or steel bowl. Add flour until you have a slightly stickier, firm dough. Shape into a ball, cover with a damp towel, and let sit for about 12 hours.
2. In the morning, spread out a sheet of parchment for a work surface. You can lightly oil it to make the dough easier to roll in a few minutes. Since you have it out already, also lightly oil your bread pan.
3. Preheat your oven to 350°F.
4. In a small bowl, combine sugar and 1 tablespoon of cinnamon. If you want a slightly sweeter bread, you can increase the sugar up to ¼ cup or a bit more. Set aside.
5. In another small bowl, combine salt and soda, making sure to break up any clumps. Sprinkle part of this and some raisins over the dough. Then fold it over, and repeat until all the salt, soda, and raisins are incorporated. This should take about 20 folds, the last few folds are just to ensure everything is fully mixed.
6. Now, carefully remove the dough from the bowl and plop it down on the parchment. With your hands (you can lightly wet or oil them first), press it out into a large rectangle. If raisins are clumped together, you can remove them and push back into the dough where needed.
7. Mix the sugar and cinnamon together in a small bowl and sprinkle the mixture across the dough. We use a spoon, but you could also use a shaker.

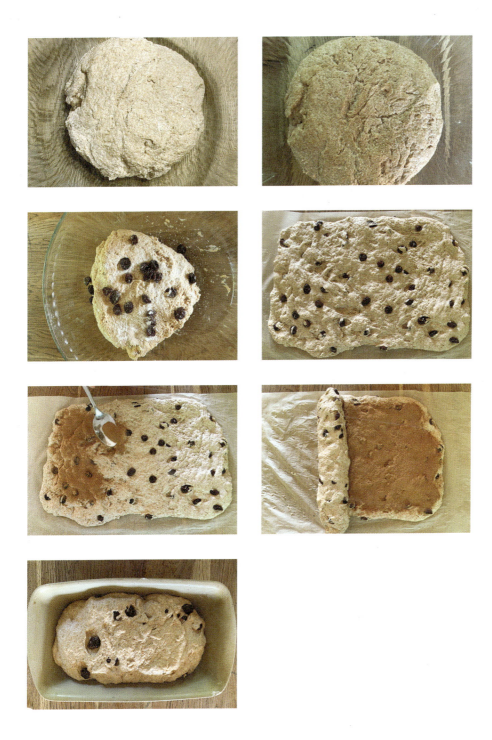

8. Start on one end, and evenly roll up the dough along the shorter side. Use your fingers to seal the loaf along the seam. For two or three mini-loaves, start on one end, and evenly roll up the dough along the longer side. Then, divide with dental floss into evenly sized loaves.
9. Gently place the dough into the bread pan. Allow to rise for about 30 minutes. Bake for about 30 minutes or until browned all around. Cool for at least 30 minutes before slicing.

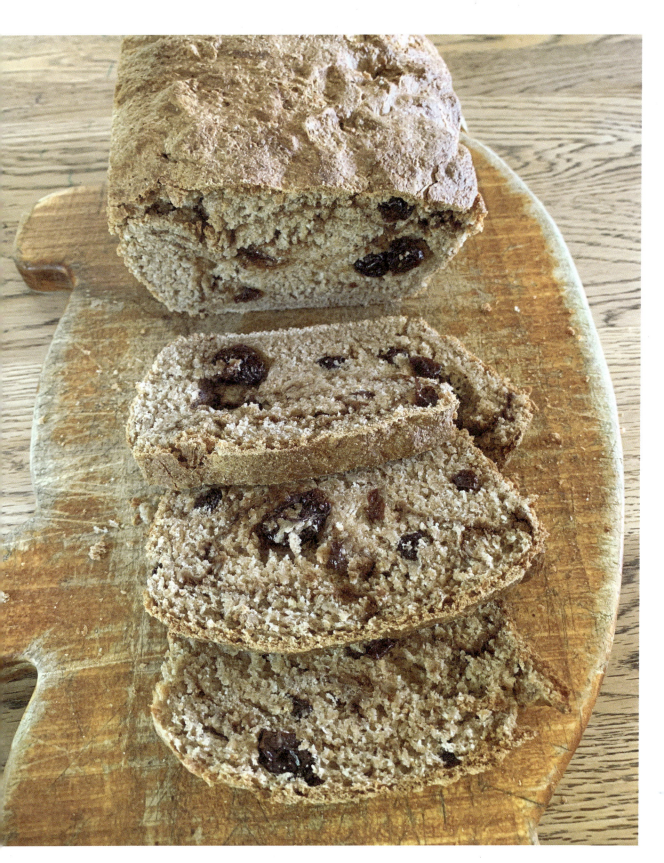

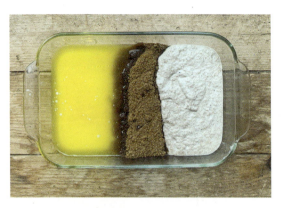
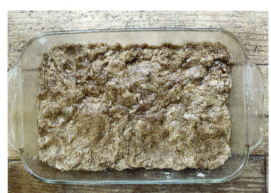
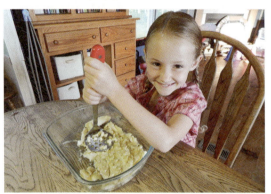
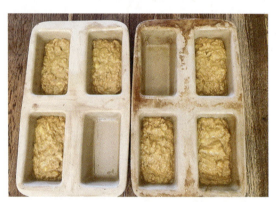
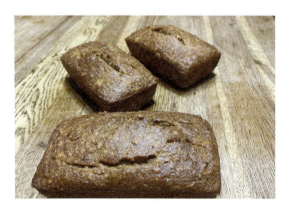
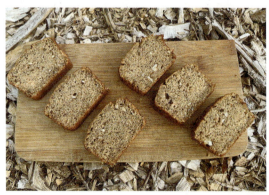

BANANA BREAD

Who hasn't bought a few too many bananas, forgotten them on some shelf or nook of counter space or the top of the refrigerator, only to rediscover them a little too late for eating? Not only are the bananas not lost but you get to turn them into a delicious snack, perfect for so many occasions that they defy easy listing!

While you can cook banana bread in regular loaf pans, we really like it in mini-loaf pans. They are like brownies; who doesn't enjoy the slightly caramelized, crunchy edges? You can also use this recipe for banana muffins with no changes needed.

This family recipe was given to Jessica's mom by a friend, and Jessica's mom gave to her, and then she has adapted it again and again. We have made it with applesauce in place of the oil, a wide array of sugars instead of white, a gluten-free flour mix in place of wheat flours, zucchini instead of bananas, and more! Here is our sourdough adaptation of an old family favorite.

1. On the night before, mix starter, butter, sugar, and flour together. It should make a thick, somewhat dry batter. Cover with a damp cloth and allow to sit until morning.
2. In the morning, preheat oven to 325°F. Combine bananas, eggs, baking soda, salt, and nuts and mix into the batter from the previous night. The batter should be quite thick, so it will take some persuasion to incorporate additional ingredients. We use the same potato/banana masher to start, and then break up any remaining doughy lumps with our hands. Banana chunks are totally fine!
3. Grease either one regular loaf or three mini-loaf pans. Pour batter into the pans. If doing three, try to keep them relatively equal. Bake the mini-loaf pans for approximately 40 minutes or a single loaf for about 1 hour, until a toothpick comes out clean from the center.
4. Cool in the pan for about 5 minutes. Then remove and finish cooling on a wire rack.

PREP TIME 15 minutes
COOK TIME 40 minutes
SERVINGS Makes one large or three small loaves

INGREDIENTS
½ cup starter
½ cup melted butter
½ cup sugar (we use coconut sugar or sucanat)
1½ cups spelt flour (or 1¼ cups whole wheat flour)
3 overripe bananas, mashed
2 eggs
1 teaspoon baking soda
½ teaspoon salt
½ cup chopped nuts (optional)

OTHER OPTIONS
This base recipe works well with many alternative ingredients, such as for pumpkin bread. We substitute 1 cup pumpkin puree for the bananas with tasty results. If using canned puree, you may need to reduce the amount by 1 tablespoon and add 1 tablespoon of water, mixed well with the puree, because it is generally so thick.

RESOURCES AND SUNDRY MATTERS

KITCHEN EQUIPMENT

It seems worth mentioning the particular brands of kitchen equipment we currently employ. Note, many, if not most, are used for other purposes beyond sourdough. Bread pans also make great meatloaf. Cookie sheets let us bake chicken nuggets, crackers, cookies, and more. Since we cook a great deal, we invest in quality and have never regretted that choice!

Cast Iron

Lodge is the most affordable and widely available cast iron brand currently on the market. There is also quite a lot of older, polished cast iron sold used online, in thrift stores and flea markets, and at yard, estate, and other such sales. This has many advantages over modern Lodge style, if you can find it. A few new companies have brought back old-style cast iron. Unfortunately, while it is amazing to cook with, the cost is generally three to four times that of a similar piece from Lodge or one of the lower-cost manufacturers. Given that cast iron will last for multiple generations if cared for properly, the difference in cost over time is small, so for some, they may well be worth the additional cost.

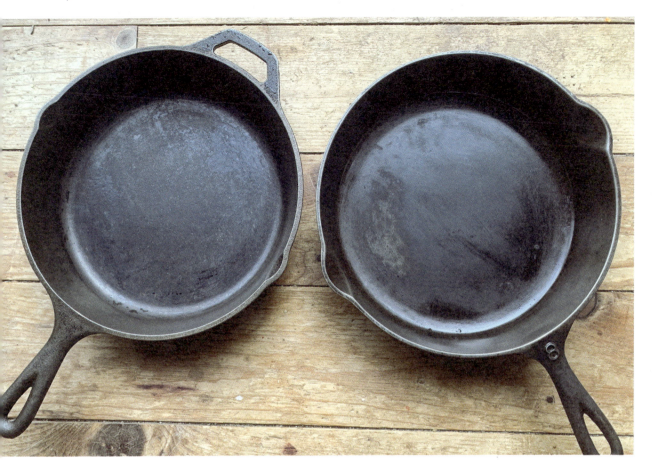

Older cast iron was finished through labor-intensive hand sanding, giving it a naturally smooth and relatively nonstick finish, unlike its modern counterparts. They are also generally far lighter than new ones.

Glass

Unfortunately, Pyrex reformulated their glass cookware in the past few years. So, older pieces are preferable, as they are far more thermal shock-resistant. Anchor, the other major brand, also performs well in our experience.

Stoneware

Soon after getting married, we purchased a large amount of Pampered Chef stoneware: regular and mini-loaf pans, muffin tins, pizza

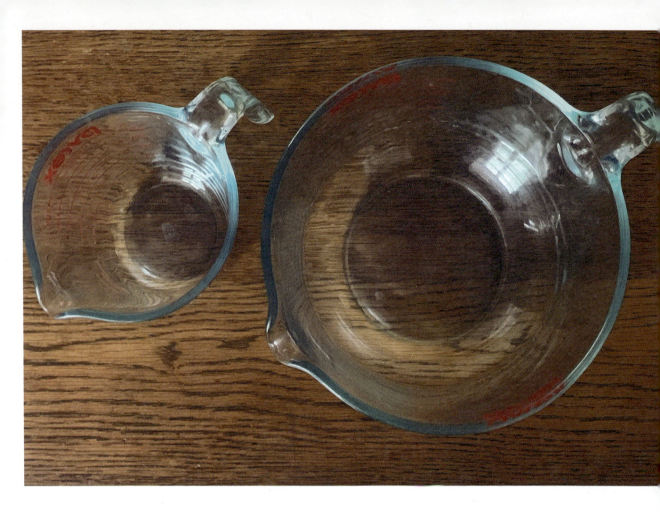

stones, bar and flat pans. Other than a few unfortunate run-ins with children (two pieces in 13 years!), most are still going strong. It was one of the best investments we made in those early days. We have cooked easily a few thousand times on the various pieces of stoneware, and they merely get better with age. We have also heard good things about Rada Cutlery stoneware.

Measuring Equipment

If it wasn't for our dear children commandeering our measuring cups and spoons for all sorts of non-kitchen permissible purposes, we would still have full sets on hand. Generally, we now find ourselves working with two or three incomplete sets of cups and spoons, accumulated over a decade. It isn't a bad idea to have more than one of the most important sizes, such as ½ teaspoon, teaspoon, and tablespoon.

Pourable measuring cups — Pyrex and OXO are the two brands we currently use — are exceptionally useful. The OXO ones are easier to use when you need precise amounts for recipes. Jessica loves the pourable Pyrex for mixing large amounts of starter, such as for pancake and waffle batter, as well as large batches of muffins and breads. We try to avoid mixing in the OXO cups since it tends to scuff and scratch the plastic, plus they are not designed for such a purpose.

Grain Mills

We have used a few grain mills over the years. Our first was so loud that the local airport asked us why we keep diverting planes to our kitchen. Our second was so heavy that our landlord was worried the floor joists would collapse without reinforcement.

Our third, which has now been with us for over twelve years, is a Family Grain Mill (previously called a Jupiter Grain Mill). Other than replacing the fuse and milling heads twice, it has performed admirably. The one drawback is that it won't create very fine flour on a first run.

Many other grain mills are available, and we hope to review a wide range in the coming years. Note that certain kitchen appliances, such as Bosch or KitchenAid mixers, often now have grain mill attachments. You can get them from both the manufacturer and other companies who have compatible mill attachments. These are often less expensive than stand-alone mills, *but* we have also seen and been told by others that they sometimes do not hold up well to consistent weekly use. It is important, if you have a lower-power appliance, to realize it may not be up to the task of grain milling on a weekly or bi-weekly basis. Such use may quickly wear down the motor or other parts, so make sure your particular model is suitable before purchasing a grain mill attachment.

ONLINE RESOURCES

There are endless websites and recipes on the internet — more than you could ever try in ten lifetimes — for those wanting to dive into the world of sourdough. We commend, in particular, the following sites to readers.

Traditional Cooking School

Wardee has numerous free recipes, articles, and videos on sourdough. For the committed person, she also offers sourdough courses, ebooks, and other resources. This is one of the few other places we have seen that uses mostly whole grains in their sourdough. https://traditionalcookingschool.com

Cultures for Health

This is the premier seller of all things microbiological — from sourdough starters, to yogurt strains from around the world, to all sorts of other fermenting friends. They also have a wide array of recipes and articles on their website. While we have had inconsistent results with some of their recipes, we often use this as a starting point for trying something new. Cultures for Health has offered a 20% discount to our readers, good for one use on any sourdough cultures or supplies. (Just use the code DIYSD20.) https://www.culturesforhealth.com

Homemade Food Junkie

This site has a great beginning artisan sourdough bread recipe as well as a whole wheat artisan sourdough recipe. It also has a wonderful video that shows all the steps for their artisan bread recipe. Books are amazing (which is why you bought this one!), but a video is so helpful when learning completely new techniques. https://www.homemadefoodjunkie.com

ABOUT THE AUTHORS

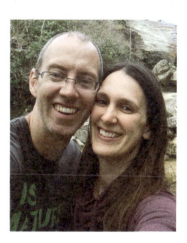

JOHN AND JESSICA Moody have been making traditional foods, including fine-tuning sourdough and other traditional whole grain preparation techniques, for over a decade. John Moody is the author of several books including *The Elderberry Book*, the founder of Whole Life Services and Whole Life Buying Club, and the former executive director of the Farm-to-Consumer Legal Defense Fund. Involved with farming, food, and homesteading, the Moody family of two old-timers and five rambunctious kids farms and homesteads on 35 acres in Kentucky.

A NOTE ABOUT THE PUBLISHER

New Society Publishers is an activist, solutions-oriented publisher focused on publishing books for a world of change. Our books offer tips, tools, and insights from leading experts in sustainable building, homesteading, climate change, environment, conscientious commerce, renewable energy, and more—positive solutions for troubled times.

We're proud to hold to the highest environmental and social standards of any publisher in North America. When you buy New Society books, you are part of the solution!

- We print all our books in North America, never overseas
- All our books are printed on 100% post-consumer recycled paper, processed chlorine free, with low-VOC vegetable-based inks (since 2002)
- Our corporate structure is an innovative employee shareholder agreement, so we're one-third employee-owned (since 2015))
- We're carbon-neutral (since 2006)
- We're certified as a B Corporation (since 2016)

At New Society Publishers, we care deeply about what we publish—but also about how we do business.

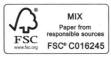

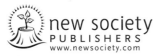

ENVIRONMENTAL BENEFITS STATEMENT

New Society Publishers saved the following resources by printing the pages of this book on chlorine free paper made with 100% post-consumer waste.

TREES	WATER	ENERGY	SOLID WASTE	GREENHOUSE GASES
23 FULLY GROWN	1,900 GALLONS	10 MILLION BTUs	80 POUNDS	9,850 POUNDS

Environmental impact estimates were made using the Environmental Paper Network Paper Calculator 4.0. For more information visit www.papercalculator.org.